STRETCHING EXERCISES FOR SENIORS OVER 60

Simple At-Home Exercises to Increase Functional Mobility, Decrease Back Pain and Injury Risk with 10-Minute Daily Workouts

STEVEN MILLS

We invite you to scan this **QR code** using the camera of your phone to access your bonus content:

SCAN THE QR CODE BELOW

You will access to **2 EBOOKS**:

1. **"Health Tips for Seniors":** The top 10 essential life tips for seniors! These strategies will help you look and feel younger in a matter of a few weeks!

2. **"Joint Health 101":** Discover the secret to healthy joints with natural home remedies, excellent exercise tips, healthy lifestyles and more

TABLE OF CONTENTS

INTRODUCTION

Welcome to *Stretching Exercises for Seniors*. Chances are that you picked this book up because you wanted to learn how to be more flexible. Regardless of how old we are, one thing we have in common is wanting to feel mobile and independent throughout our daily tasks.

You might notice that you are not nearly as flexible as you once were. Perhaps things, such as bending down, getting up from the floor, or reaching for items on a high shelf have become increasingly complex. Maybe you have noticed that your joints struggle to straighten or move easily.

Realistically, we are all aging, and there is nothing you can do to prevent your daily trips around the sun and moon from stopping the process, but you can work on your muscles, joints, tendons, and ligaments by stretching so that you can continue to move.

Flexibility is essential for everything in life, but it is crucial for seniors. This does not mean you should turn yourself into a pretzel or do full splits like a gymnast. It means you should move without restriction or pain from stiff joints and tense muscles. However, an aging body means that flexibility will decrease, especially when we forget to take care of our muscles so we can move easily. Unfortunately, as we age, our joints' range of motion decreases. As a result, most of us have lost or will lose between 25% and 30% by the time we are 70. You may even find that some of your joints are more affected than others. Losing flexibility in our bodies is due to the increased rigidity of the ligaments and tendons around the joints.

Within our skin and bones, we have connective tissue, which are the collagen fibers that make up our tendons and ligament structures around our joints. When changes occur, our tendons and ligaments become stiff, preventing us from moving swiftly. In addition, the elastin content, which contributes to our structure's elasticity, also reduces its stretching ability, making some areas tense or stiff.

The good news is that exercising can slow your body's aging process and help you maintain better flexibility. In addition, it aligns with working out regularly to help prevent health problems, such as diabetes and heart disease. Remaining flexible as you age benefits you by reducing injury, maintaining your balance, and continuing to have a good range of motion.

HOW TO DETERMINE YOUR FLEXIBILITY

Being flexible means you can achieve a range of motion without pain. Try this exercise to determine your flexibility level:

Sit in a chair with your legs extended out in front of you and your toes facing the ceiling. You will want to ensure your legs are on a diagonal from your hips. If you are on the shorter side, it's recommended that you roll a towel or a blanket to place your heels on. Ensure that your knees are soft and not locked out.

1. Inhale as you slowly reach forward toward your toes as far as you can until you feel a stretch. You can expect to feel a stretch in your lower and upper back, hamstrings, and calves. Be sure only to reach until you feel mild discomfort. You do not want to try and push past any pain, as this can injure you.
2. Exhale and drop your head to reach the best results of the stretch.
3. Inhale to return to the starting position.

If you can touch your toes, that's great! However, keep in mind that stretching daily, or at least a few times a week, will help you maintain that flexibility as you get older. However, if you find your flexibility is not where you would like it to be, don't worry. There are several ways to increase your flexibility and the range of motion in your joints.

Regardless of where you are physically, know that you can improve your flexibility and range of motion in your joints regardless of age.

THE BENEFITS OF MAINTAINING FLEXIBILITY

When you work on flexibility, you will find that your posture and balance improve, lessening the chances of injury. Remember, your level of flexibility or fitness does not matter because there is always time to start today and the opportunity to learn the skills to live a healthier life.

How Do You Decide When to Stretch?

There are two ways you can think about when to stretch. First, if you are an active senior who routinely jogs, walks, or participates in other forms of exercise, you might choose to stretch at a different time compared to someone who may be less active. If you are more active, your best time to stretch is after your workout, which will be explained in a deeper context in Chapter 8.

Second, you can stretch at any point during the day if you are a less active senior. However, the best recommendation is to stretch in the mornings or evenings. In Chapter 9, you will find a workout plan best-suited for this purpose.

Always remember that stretching muscles does not count as a warm-up. Getting your heart rate and body temperature up is essential to getting the most out of your stretching, especially if you are active.

In this book, you are going to learn:
- The importance of stretching and why it is going to help you
- How to stretch safely
- Stretches you can do for a warm-up

- Various stretches for your lower and upper body
- Stretches you can do if you suffer from arthritis, sciatica, or nerve pain
- Equipment you can use for stretching
- Post-workout stretches

This book will give you all the tools and stretches you need to remain limber and regain your flexibility. Your only action is to put in the effort and stay consistently on the path. In time, you will become more flexible. Whether you take a handful of the stretches in this book to incorporate into your routine or follow one of the five plans outlined in Chapter 9 is entirely up to you, as everything you want to accomplish is in your control.

My one hope for you is that you finish this book knowing that you can regain your flexibility so that you can play with your grandchildren or do daily tasks with few issues. Let's begin.

CHAPTER ONE
THE IMPORTANCE OF STRETCHING

It's no secret that aging affects our bodies and that maintaining our overall mobility can be difficult. Many people age well and can remain active, alert, and energized throughout their lives; they might even feel younger than they are.

However, others might feel like they are slowing due to osteoporosis, osteoarthritis, or arthritis, all of which minimize their ability to participate in most activities.

Stretching is an excellent way to help ease those aches, loosen muscles, and relax joints. This is why it is essential to know how to be proactive and take steps to counterbalance the aging effects so you can feel vibrant, young, and independent, no matter your age.

THE PHYSICAL EFFECTS OF AGING

Here are some of the effects you may experience:

- Aging muscles
- Aging bones
- Aging joints

As our muscles age, they start to shrink and lose their mass. It is a natural process, but could be sped up if you tend to live a more sedentary than active lifestyle. Our heart, our most important muscle, also begins to slow with age, reducing the ability to move blood more fluidly through the body. This is likely the culprit if you find yourself easily fatigued or take longer to recover. However, you are encouraged to contact your doctor if you think it is something else. Remember, listening to your body is essential, especially regarding heart health.

As we get older, our bones begin to undergo a process of absorption and formation. Unfortunately, during this period, it has been found that the balance between the bones starts to decrease in bone tissues, making them more fragile. When your bone mass depletes, you are more likely to develop osteoporosis. This condition can lead to a hump in your back, also known as a dowager's hump. This is all due to a series of crash fractures in the vertebrae.

Lastly, our skeletal structure has ligaments and cartilage, the connective tissues between the bones. When the elasticity reduces in the ligaments, mobility is impacted. In addition, there is less water content in the cartilage, which leaves your joints more open to stress that, down the road, can lead to arthritis. Overall, if you are not using specific joints, chances are you will see them impacted more than others which is why it is necessary to stretch all extremities, so one is not overcompensating for another.

Short-Term Effects of Stretching

The short-term effects of stretching include:

- Injury prevention
- Mindfulness and stress release
- Quick recovery
- Pain relief
- Preparation for the next day's activities

Injury Prevention

Some injuries can come from a muscle imbalance. When our muscles are tight, they tend to use another muscle to compensate and provide an equal distribution. Unfortunately, the compensation will force stress onto the joint and surrounding structure. By stretching, you will help balance out the muscle and the fascia (the thin tissues that hold everything together). In turn, the tight muscle that was causing the poor distribution will be released.

Mindfulness and Stress Release

When it comes to mindfulness, it's sometimes easy to forget that our mind and body are connected, but they are! These connections have proven that our mind feels stress when we are physically tense. From there, the brainwaves will shift from a relaxed state to an anxious one; think of the fight or flight response. When we are prepared for danger, our anxious energy tightens up the muscles and causes our brain to be more alert. If you are less tense, you will be more focused. Stretching, therefore, can give you a sense of clarity and better well-being.

In addition to being mindful, stretching allows you to find yourself in the present moment. Connecting to your mind allows you to become aware of the more minor details that your brain will absorb and then send the messages elsewhere and allow you to live fully.

Quick Recovery

For the more active seniors, stretching after a workout gives them a quicker recovery since the circulation and blood flow release lactic acid build-up in their muscles. It is necessary to note here, however, that recovery is not solely about recovering from the physical activity or workout you have just completed. It's also about getting the benefits, too. For example, feeling the burn from a workout is great because you know you have worked a specific set of muscle groups, such as your legs, in your training; you want to feel that burn to know they are activating in particular exercises. However, a misaligned muscle pulling a joint is not good pain. This indicates that you either did not set yourself up correctly for a repetition in an exercise or may have an existing injury. In that case, be mindful because it can mean you must rest the area.

Pain Relief

Stretching is meant to help decompress the muscles, so we can continue to live pain-free while we perform everyday tasks such as walking. Even if the muscle pain is present the following day, stretching will continue to help release the build-up to help you feel good. However, if it irritates an area, stop because pushing through the pain will not have the benefits you want and could cause injury.

In addition, about 33.6% of seniors are estimated to be affected by osteoarthritis, which is why you want to ensure you have all the benefits of stretching in your daily routine.

Preparing for the Next Day's Activities

Stretching also helps decrease compression, which affects your range of motion and impacts your next workout or physical activity. Imagine yourself as a machine. Machines need to have moving parts to function. Likewise, your body is a machine, and stretching continues to help you move efficiently and pain-free every day, just as grease will keep a machine's gears moving fluidly.

Some of these short-term effects also will flow into the long-term effects as well. Keep in mind, everything is connected in one way or another.

Long-Term Effects of Stretching

The long-term effects of stretching include:

- Posture
- Flexibility and range of motion
- Body awareness
- Balance
- Fitness capability
- Weight loss and control

Posture

Remember when our parents told us not to slouch at the dinner table? Was it an old-fashioned idea or is it really important? In this case, it's the latter. The spine is our central piece and helps lift you up. Our neurological responses also occur in the spinal cord, so your spine is your connector hub to everything in your body and mind.

Your immune and nervous systems are within the spinal cord, so you want those to function correctly. Additionally, most of our major organs are housed in our ribcage, which is also attached to the spine.

If you have poor posture, your body's ability to react to internal and external factors and your desire to live pain-free can be impacted. Clarke (2014) defines poor posture as our spine being "positioned in unnatural positions, in which the curves are emphasized." The results from the emphasized curves mean the "joints, muscles, and vertebrae" are put into stressful positions (Clarke, 2014). Other contributions to poor posture decrease the body's water content in the connective tissues. When the fluid reduces, the elasticity and flexibility go with it.

Therefore, adding stretching into your daily routine, or at least three to four times a week, can positively impact your posture and reduce pain in other areas.

Additionally, a good posture helps with your breathing, digestive system, and heart health, so it is much more than just keeping your head high and straight. Some even believe that a good posture is one of the best anti-aging tonics!

Flexibility and Range of Motion

Without flexibility, you do not have a range of motion. Stiff bodies are stringent, and they don't operate well. Life is meant to be about movement, whether in sport, regular exercise such as walking, or in an artistic form like dance or Tai Chi. Lack of mobility leads to aging and can make us feel older than our chronological age. Be patient with yourself, though.

Body Awareness

Knowing how your body is feeling is a skill set anyone can learn, but it takes time. For example, as we stretch, we understand what feels good for us through the movement of the stretch. So as we learn the skill set, we are more in tune with our body, what it likes, what it doesn't like, what it needs, and what it doesn't need. As you already know, connecting with your body can help you identify and correct the problems, preventing further damage or injury.

Balance

When houses or condos are built, they are built on a foundation and with balance and symmetry. If they lack a solid foundation, balance, and symmetry, their chances of crumbling are high. Our bodies are no different, creating the big concern of falling among seniors. A tight muscle on one side is going to impact the other side. Studies have found that stretching regularly contributes to remaining balanced and can help prevent falls that can be severe or worse.

Fitness Capabilities

We discussed earlier in the chapter how our loss of muscle mass can impact the mechanics of our body. Stretching will help out smaller muscles that don't always work activated while helping the larger muscles operate better. In addition, long-term stretching means you can continue exercising into your later years without feeling any limitations or pain.

Weight Loss and Control

If weight loss is a goal for you, you may not even think of stretching as part of your journey, but it is tied into it. The relationship between our muscle mass and weight control is hardwired. When you stretch, you open up and release muscles that are not activating because they are tight. The more muscles you work, the more they can burn and fuel the mitochondria. The more mitochondria you have, the more unnecessary calories you will burn.

Regardless of your needs when it comes to stretching, you can see why it is an essential part of your day. Let's learn about the different kinds of stretching.

Three Kinds of Stretching

When it comes to stretching, there are three different types:

- Dynamic
- Static
- Proprioceptive neuromuscular facilitation

What Is Dynamic Stretching?

Dynamic stretching means that you are moving your body through a movement to achieve the stretch. For example, you typically use dynamic stretching as part of your warm-up routine. Additionally, dynamic stretching is known to increase your blood flow and boost your energy due to the movement portion of the stretches.

What Is Static Stretching?

Static stretching requires you to stretch and hold your muscle's position as far as it can go for a minimum amount of time, with repetitions typically between one and three times.

Chapters 3 to 5 will cover a variety of static and dynamic stretches you can do. However, we will not cover stretching involving proprioceptive neuromuscular facilitation, as this type of stretching must be under the guidance of a physiotherapist.

From this chapter, you should take away that:

- Stretching is essential to help you live a pain-free and mobile life
- The short- and long-term effects of stretching when you incorporate them into your daily or weekly routines
- The two kinds of stretching that will help you toward your stretching goals

CHAPTER TWO
STRETCHING SAFELY

The benefits of physical activity have long been connected to living a longer, fuller life. However, as we slow down, some of us are more likely to shy away from being active. We tend to forget that every activity we do, even as simple as picking something off the floor, relies on movement and how easy the action is.

Exercising helps keep you healthy; stretching contributes to less tense muscles so you can continue to move. There are always safety precautions to be aware of, especially if you are older or have chronic conditions.

HOW TO ENSURE YOU STRETCH SAFELY

Perhaps you have felt tense or stiff in your joints for some time, and you might feel eager to jump right in on improving your flexibility. However, rushing can lead to injury, so the first tip is to be patient with yourself.

As with any body movement, you might be tempted to stretch immediately, especially if you are going to do a moderate to vigorous activity, but you must warm up first. Think of your muscle like it is taffy. Taffy needs to be warm for it to stretch. Our muscles are very much the same, and they move better when they are warm. Conversely, you can risk injuring yourself if you perform stretches while your muscles are cold. Warming up can be as little as marching in place with your arms swinging or dancing to a few songs to going for a brisk walk around the block. As long as you move to get your heart moving and body temperature up, your muscles will react better to the stretches.

Posture is also essential, whether moving, standing, or sitting. This means ensuring that your shoulders are back and down, maintaining a neutral position of your hips and spine and engaging your core. An excellent stretching posture will give you better flexibility and a reduced risk of injury when stretching your tight muscles. Breathing is natural, but we sometimes forget it when doing strenuous exercises or stretching. When stretching, you need to be mindful of breathing because it allows you to find movement through the full range of motion, regardless of whether the stretch is dynamic or static. When you hold your breath, you deny your muscles the oxygen they need to move or stretch correctly. So instead, relax into your stretches with easy breathing. Feel the deep inhale and exhale in your lungs and diaphragm. Stretch to the point of mild discomfort. You never want to stretch to the point that it causes you pain. If you find that a stretch is hurting, stop and reset. If you repeat the stretch and it is still causing you pain, avoid it and find out from your doctor or physiotherapist if the move is right for you or if you are doing it correctly. You also want to ensure that you are not stretching injuries; you want those to heal. If the injury is recent, give yourself a minimum of six weeks for recovery before attempting to stretch.

As you stretch a specific muscle group, pay attention to it. The focus will allow you to learn which side is tighter. Your goal is to balance it out to prevent overcompensation.

You will also want to avoid ballistic stretching, where you bounce to push your body past a normal range of motion. This type of stretching requires extra force, which may result in a strained or pulled muscle.

Lastly, be sure to wear comfortable clothes that will not restrict your movements.

Chronic Conditions

When we experience pain, it is an indicator of our brain pointing to an injury, illness, or maybe the work of a good training session; in that case, the pain is often seen as good pain.

It is labeled chronic pain or condition in other situations where the pain does not subside after a minimum of three to six months.

Other chronic pain or conditions include:
- Complex regional pain syndrome causes severe pain in your hands, feet, legs, or arms.

- Fibromyalgia is where there is extensive pain in muscles and bones.
- Chronic fatigue syndrome, also known as myalgic encephalomyelitis, is where extreme exhaustion is felt in addition to severe muscle and bone pain.
- Myofascial pain syndrome creates knots and tightness, making movements difficult.

It is not entirely understood what causes the above chronic conditions. Sometimes, it can result from a forceful trauma, a stressful event, a virus, or a pulled muscle, but the root cause is hard to identify in each case.

If you have any of these conditions, it is imperative to be mindful of your body and listen to its needs so that you don't hurt yourself. Follow the less is more rule, and if you need to sit instead of stand, do so.

Another important reminder is that stretching is an excellent way to improve flexibility. Still, it is not intended to be a treatment or cure for ailments or medical conditions, nor does it replace advice from a professional.

Before beginning any exercise program, check with your doctor or physiotherapist to determine the suitable stretches, especially if you have arthritis, balance issues, osteoporosis, or a hip or knee replacement. Depending on the severity of your chronic condition, you might need to avoid specific stretches or movements altogether.

CHAPTER THREE
WARM-UP STRETCHES

It's an amusing concept, but when we look at our grandkids, they seem to be able to run full tilt and not feel it in their bodies later.

But, as older adults, we feel the repercussions, and it has everything to do with not warming up.

As we hit young and middle age, physical activities or workouts are important, and for seniors, it's essential.

However, when you think about warming up before a workout, it is more than just a few simple stretches.

However, you should never jump right into stretching with cold muscles as they won't be ready to move and lengthen, and you could hurt yourself by pulling the muscle.

Thus, it's essential to warm our body temperature to ensure our lungs and heart are prepared for exercise and stretching.

But, there are also debates on if it is of use or not, so let's debunk stretching first.

THE BIG DEBATE ON STRETCHING

Exercising alone presents challenges, and, to be honest, there is conflicting information on how to best create a routine that works for you. Realistically, we are all different, and not every exercise or workout plan is one size fits all. For example, stretching is one area of debate, and that many cannot seem to find common ground. Some say to nix the stretching, static stretching more specifically, because it is a waste of time. But on the other hand, some swear that stretching can help ward off injuries.

Realistically, stretching is not as easy as it might sound, and each one benefits a particular part of your workout. However, as you understand now, stretching is an excellent practice to incorporate into your routines, even if you are not overly active. When we aren't flexible, our mobility becomes impacted, and, just like running full tilt as an older person, we feel the repercussions.

When the word stretch is mentioned, most people think of static stretching. That might be holding a quadricep stretch and holding it for 30 seconds or bending down to touch your toes, for example. However, static stretching alone is not enough.

WHY ISN'T STRETCHING ALONE ENOUGH?

At one point, many believed stretching before exercise was like dating before getting engaged, a vital step before the more significant events. In addition, athletes were once told to stretch before they fatigued their muscles to avoid a severe pull or injury. Unfortunately, that information and advice were not the best.

Studies have found that stretching, more specifically static stretching, before a strenuous activity impacts your body's overall performance. The research, which studied multiple runners, jumpers, and weightlifters, found that they ran slower, jumped lower, and lifted weaker when they stretched before the strenuous activity. What you can take away from this is that, regardless of what you once were told, whether it brings you back to gym class or not, you should not perform a static stretch before you exercise. You need to warm your muscles first to gain the benefits of a static stretch. Remember the taffy concept from Chapter 2? Picture your muscles like taffy: To lengthen them, they need to be warm. That is not to say that static stretching isn't good for you; it should not be your go-to for stretching right away and is more beneficial at the end of your workout.

Here is what you can do to start stretching, though: light cardio. A small amount of cardio will help your heart rate, allowing more oxygen to move through your circulation. This is all due to your blood vessels dilating to ensure that your muscles get a good supply of oxygen. When oxygen is delivered to your muscles, you will have increased movement efficiency and optimal flexibility. In addition, warm-ups reduce tension and stress so that you are mentally prepared for the activity you are about to do.

How to Warm Up Before an Exercise

If you are preparing to do a light workout, your warm-up should take around 10 minutes, involving some light aerobic activity and dynamic stretching. Here are some ideas to get you started:

- Fast-paced walking
- Climbing and descending the stairs
- Quick side-steps
- Marching or jogging on the spot
- Jumping jacks
- Step-ups on an aerobic step or balance pad

After the Light Cardio Warm-up

After you have spent 10 minutes warming up, move into some dynamic stretching. Dynamic stretching will have you move your muscles through the movement. As such, your body will be able to reach its optimal; movement during activities such as playing tennis, going for a hike, lifting heavier objects or weights, or general exercise. The actions should align with the activity you are going to do. For example, if you intend to do heavy weightlifting with your legs, your dynamic movement should involve dynamic leg stretches.

Warm-Up Stretching Exercises

After you have spent about 10 minutes doing light aerobic cardio, you can now begin utilizing some of these warm-up stretching exercises.

WAIST TWISTS

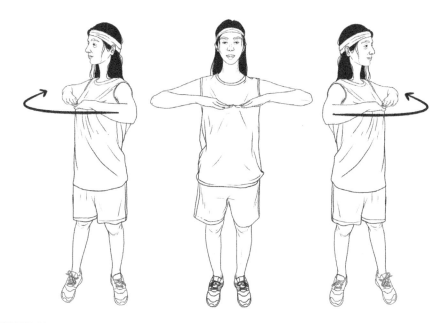

INTRODUCTION

This warm-up stretching exercise is fun! The twisting motion in this exercise will help open your hips up and loosen your arms as they flap against your body with each twist.

For this exercise, you will want to stand straight with your feet slightly wider than your hips and your arms hanging by your sides.

INSTRUCTIONS

1. Keeping your head, shoulders, and upper back facing the front, turn your hips to the left. The rotation should be minimal, so be sure not to lift your right foot in the twist.

2. Twist to the right side next, keeping the rotation minimal.

3. Repeat in each direction at least five times.

As you continue, you may begin to include your spine, shoulders, and head in the movement. Repeat the motion for two minutes.

TORSO TWIST

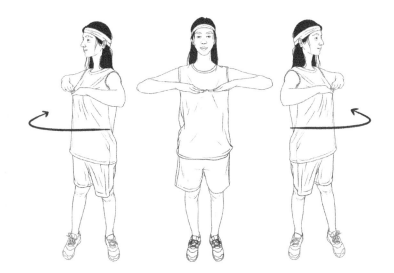

INTRODUCTION

The previous exercise warmed up your hips. The torso twist will warm your torso and prepare your body to do flexion, extension, forward, and backbend movements. The torso twist will also help build a stronger core and back muscles, improving mobility. The primary areas that the torso twist will affect are your abs and obliques. In addition, your quads, rhomboids, deltoids, glutes, and abductors will also be affected during torso twists. This warm-up exercise is not recommended in a chair as it could cause strain or injury.

INSTRUCTIONS

1. Stand straight with your legs slightly wider than the hips. Keep your knees soft and ankles under your knees.
2. Place your hands on your hips to feel how they twist.
3. Inhale to lengthen your spine.
4. Exhale and rotate your torso to the left, going only as far as you can without significantly turning your hips. Ideally, you only want to rotate about 40% of the way.
5. Twist back to the right.

↻ Repeat the twisting motion about 5-10 times in each direction.

SHOULDER BLADE SQUEEZES

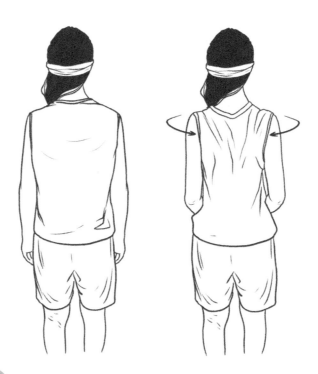

INTRODUCTION

This exercise brings attention to drawing and squeezing your shoulder blades together. It works explicitly on the rhomboid muscles and can help the shoulder and upper limb stability. You want to keep your shoulders stable to do every movement, such as pushing, pulling, and holding objects. This exercise can also help with your posture to help avoid rounded shoulders.

INSTRUCTIONS

1. Stand or sit straight with your arms by your side.
2. Squeeze your shoulder blades together as you pull your arms and elbows back.
3. Release and repeat 10-20 times.

LEG SWINGS

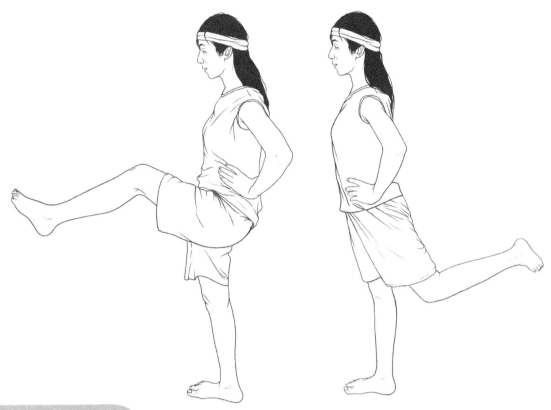

INTRODUCTION

The purpose of leg swings is to help warm up and stretch your hip muscles and hip joints, preventing any injuries. This exercise also helps to reduce any pain you might have in the area. For this exercise, you will need enough space for your leg to swing forward and backward easily. You will also need a chair, wall, table, or countertop for support.

INSTRUCTIONS

1. Standing sideways to your chair with your right leg to the outside.
2. Begin to swing your leg forward to the height that is comfortable for you.
3. Swing your leg backward as high as you can go. You are likely not lifting it nearly as high as you did in the front.
4. Repeat 10-15 times, and then turn to swing your left leg.

ANKLE CIRCLES

INTRODUCTION

The ankle circle is a dynamic stretch that will open your ankle joints and release stress and tension. You will find that the exercise will improve your ankle's flexibility while warming up your calves, feet, and ankles.

You can do this exercise either seated or standing. If you are standing, try not to use a chair, table, countertop, or wall for support to test and challenge your balance.

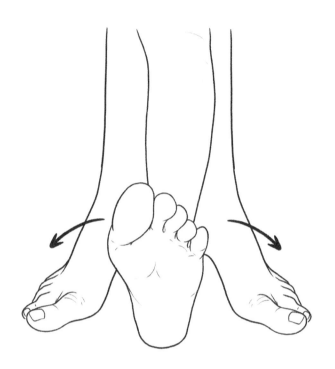

INSTRUCTIONS

1. Bring your right ankle a few inches off of the ground.
2. Begin to make clockwise circles with your ankle for 10 rotations.
3. Switch to go counterclockwise.

↻ For an added challenge to this exercise, sit in a chair, extend both legs out in front of you, and try rotating them outwards simultaneously and then inwards.

WINDMILL

INTRODUCTION

The windmill is a full-body movement that can help strengthen your core, shoulders, and hips. You allow your muscles to learn how to become more flexible and strong as they move in various directions. In addition, your spine will get some more rotation. What is more beneficial about the windmill is that you work on each side of your body one at a time, which can help you identify any imbalances you might have.

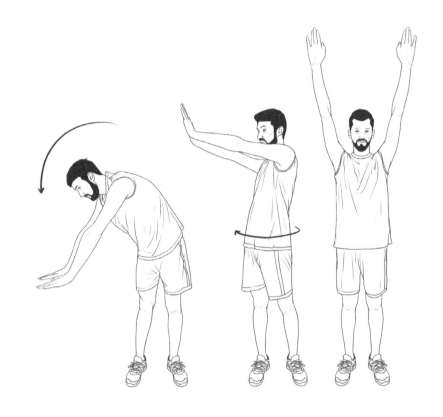

INSTRUCTIONS

1. Stand with your legs slightly wider than shoulder width.
2. Let your arms loosely hang by your sides and relax your shoulders.
3. Inhale and sweep your arms out and over your head like a windmill turning its blades.
4. Stop when you reach the top and arch your spine as you reach for the sky.
5. Exhale to bend toward the floor with your arms hanging in front of you.

↻ Repeat 5-10 times in each direction.

CHAPTER FOUR

LOWER BODY STRETCHES

The lower body is the most critical area for mobility and includes your calves, hip flexors, hamstrings, pelvis, and quadriceps.

Since our legs are the largest extremities on our body, they require the most stretches for the full benefits.

However, did you know that about half of us spend about six to seven hours sitting daily? The amount of time we sit opens us to a range of short- and long-term effects on our health and body.

It isn't because we are lazy. On the contrary, most sedentary activities, such as crafts or working, require sitting for an extended period.

In addition, most of us are either working at a computer or driving for short or long periods to run errands, so after a busy day, it feels good to curl up in your favorite spot on the couch or in a chair to unwind with a book or a television show.

Not that any of these activities are invaluable to living a vibrant life, but almost everything we do requires sitting at some point.

HOW SITTING AFFECTS YOUR BODY

Although sitting for a long time is sometimes unavoidable, you want to ensure that you get up and move so that your risk of developing a health condition can be minimized or avoided. Here you will learn about some of the adverse side effects that sitting too long can do to you.

Chronic Illness

The longer you are sitting, the higher your risk is of developing a chronic illness such as:

- Diabetes: Sitting for long periods can contribute to your body resisting insulin and increasing blood sugar levels.
- Heart disease: Some studies have found that sitting is linked to heart disease later in life.
- Cancer: It's not understood why or what the correlation is, but studies have found that people who sat for longer periods than those who did not were at a higher risk of developing certain types of cancers

Vein Disease

When we sit for a long time, our blood circulation becomes negatively impacted. For example, have you ever noticed that your legs felt puffy and heavy after being on a plane? Chances are, you probably did not get up often to move around. What happened was that pressure began to build up in your lower body's veins and caused blood to pool in your legs. Unfortunately, when you are not taking the time to get up and move around, whether or not on a plane, you open the risk of developing vein disease, which can become problematic and more serious over time.

Varicose Veins

Varicose veins are where the pooling of blood creates pressure in a vein that can cause it to bulge into a varicose vein. The condition is not deadly, but it can indicate a more serious vein problem and may cause discomfort or pain.

Deep Vein Thrombosis

Deep vein thrombosis occurs when you sit a long time, especially in a car or airplane. This condition can cause a blood clot to form in your legs. This disease is serious and can cause a pulmonary embolism if left untreated.

Weight Gain

When you are sitting, you burn fewer calories than working out routinely. This is due to your muscles being inactive and not processing the food that you eat. Instead, your body keeps the fats and sugars in your system, with both contributing to weight gain.

Digestive Issues

In this era, so many adults are busy that they often eat lunch at their desks. However, sitting and eating causes the food to compress and slows the digestive process. Without movements, you are more at risk of feeling bloated and constipated, or you may experience cramping that makes you less productive.

Poor Posture

We have already touched on poor posture. You may start your day by sitting up straight with your shoulders back and down and your core engaged, but as you get busy, you forget. However, a desk or table's height can also contribute to poor posture. If it is too low, you are more likely to hunch over your desk or table subconsciously.

Muscle Weakness

Muscles are more likely to become tenser and stiffer over long periods of sitting. Over time, our core will also become weaker, leading to poor posture. Your hips, glutes, and leg muscles will also become tighter from inactivity. You do not want this since your legs are the foundation for standing and balance. With an impacted range of motion, the risk of falling is higher, which is a considerable concern in older adults.

HINTS YOU NEED TO STRETCH YOUR LOWER BODY

If you are more active and find that you become injured frequently, are you ensuring you are warming up and cooling down properly? If not, this is your first sign that you need to stretch more. Even if you are not exercising frequently, you might find that daily activities, such as walking, can become impacted when you are less flexible. General aches and pains are another sign that you need to be stretching. Things you can watch out for include feeling stiffer when you wake up in the morning or if moving is taking a little bit longer, which are clear indicators that you might need to stretch your lower body.

Another sign is an extended period of achiness following exercise. Remember, stretching improves your circulation and blood flow. So not only does it help prepare your muscles for a workout, but it also helps repair the tissue damage afterward.

Dynamic Lower Body Stretches

In this part, you will learn different dynamic lower body stretches you can incorporate into your routine. Remember to listen to your body and its needs. If something does not feel right, stop.

SEATED KNEE-TO-CHEST STRETCH

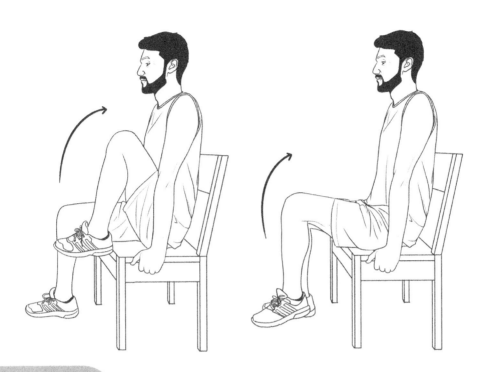

INTRODUCTION

This exercise is important to maintain and improve the mobility in your hips and knees by stretching the correlating joints. In addition, this stretch will benefit your lower back's flexibility. You will need a chair for this stretch.

INSTRUCTIONS

1. Sit comfortably on the edge of your chair not too far forward.
2. Bring your right knee up.
3. Use your right hand to gently pull your knee to your chest .
4. Once you feel a comfortable stretch, hold it for 20 to 30 seconds.
5. Release and repeat on the other side.

↻ Repeat this stretch 10 times.

HIP FLEXOR STRETCH

INTRODUCTION

If you find that you have a stiff or tense lower back, tight hip flexors are likely the root of the problem. The hip flexors are a set of muscles found in the front of your upper thighs and support a variety of movements. Thus, you should be doing the hip flexor stretch for many reasons. It helps to improve your hip mobility, alleviates pain, increases flexibility, and helps to improve your posture to continue moving without issue or pain.

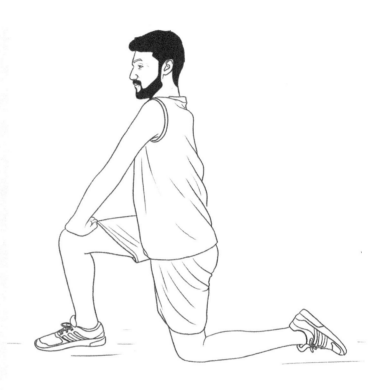

INSTRUCTIONS

1. On the floor, start with your right leg in a 90-degree position and your left leg bent behind you.
2. Inhale and lean forward. You can place your hands on your knee for support or on either side of your foot on the floor.
3. Hold for 10-15 seconds.
4. Return to the starting position.

Repeat on the right leg five times before switching to the left side.

WALKING KNEE HUGS

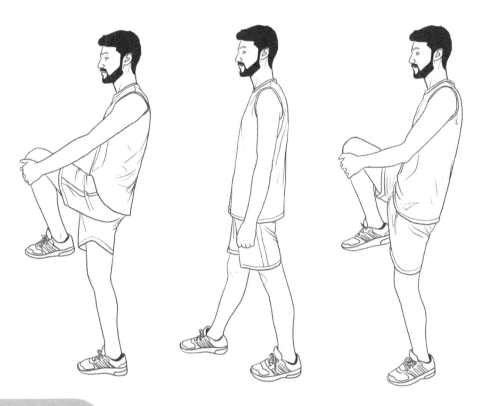

INTRODUCTION

The walking knee hug is an exercise that will warm up and stretch your hips, glutes, quads, hamstrings, and calves. This exercise will also challenge your balance as you switch from standing on one leg to the other.

INSTRUCTIONS

1. Start by standing with your feet together.

2. Bring your right leg up with your knee bent and simultaneously grab your knee with both hands to pull it up higher. You should feel your glute stretching as you lean forward.

3. Put your right leg down and immediately step up with your left leg and repeat the same actions.

4. Keep walking forward and switching legs, doing this exercise for 30 seconds.

WALKING LUNGES

INTRODUCTION

This variation of the lunge strengthens your legs in addition to your core, hips, and glutes. Your balance is going to be tested as you walk forward. Make sure you have enough space to take at least 10 steps.

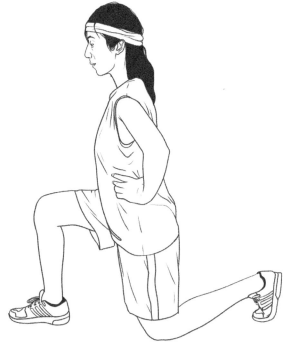

INSTRUCTIONS

1. Stand on one side of the room with your legs shoulder-width apart. Place your hands on your hips.

2. Step forward with your right leg with your weight pushing into your heel as you bend your right knee, lowering so that your quad and left shin are parallel to the floor.

3. Hold for a second or two and then repeat with the left side stepping forward.

↻ Continue until you have reached the end of the room. Then, turn around to return to the opposite direction repeating two to three times each way.

BACK EXTENSIONS

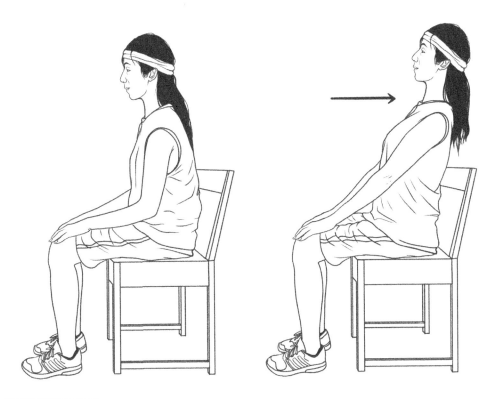

INTRODUCTION

Back extensions are an excellent exercise to help strengthen the muscles in your lower back. You will benefit from this exercise as it will help reduce lower back pain, strengthen your posterior chain, improve your hip flexion, and improve your posture. You will need a chair for this exercise.

INSTRUCTIONS

1. Sit tall in your chair with your shoulders down and back.
2. Bring your arms to the small of your back and lean into your hands, creating an arch in your spine.
3. Hold for 5-10 seconds and then release.

↻ Repeat 10 times.

Static Lower Body Stretches

Although it is tempting to leap right into these stretches before a workout, it is best practice to do them after since your body is already warm. As always, listen to your body for cues if the stretch feels right to you or not.

BUTTERFLY STRETCH

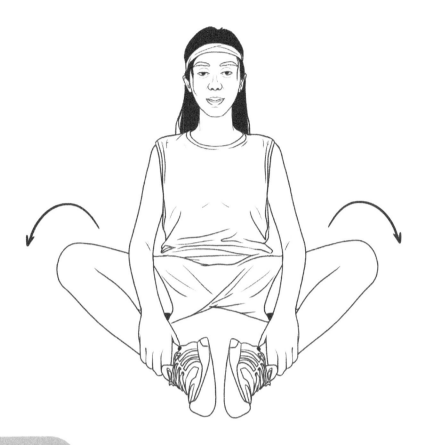

The butterfly stretch is excellent for your adductor muscles and serves as a hip opener.

INSTRUCTIONS

1. Sit on the floor and bring the bottoms of your feet together with your heels as close to your pelvis as possible.
2. Bring your hands to the heart center in a yoga prayer pose. You have the option to place them on your knees as well.
3. Hold for 15 seconds.

↻ Slowly extend your legs and bring them back to repeat two more times.

LUMBAR FLEXION STRETCH

INTRODUCTION

The lumbar flexion stretch is a simple stretch to help with lumbar mobility. This stretch is beneficial if you have lower back pain. In addition, this exercise may be beneficial if you are recovering from a herniated disk or a bulging disk. However, caution is advised because the stretch could worsen your condition, so you should check with your physiotherapist before proceeding.

You can do this in your bed, but the best results for the stretch are on the floor.

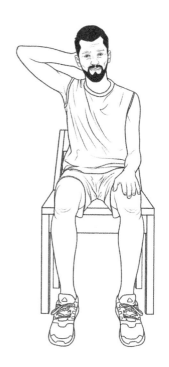
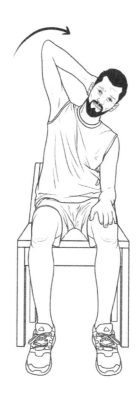

INSTRUCTIONS

1. Lie on your back and bend your knees, so your feet are flat on the floor.
2. Bring both knees up to your chest, hugging them or grabbing your knees with your hands. If either is uncomfortable, you have the option to hold your thighs underneath your knees.
3. Gently pull your knees toward your chest and hold for three to five seconds.
4. Slowly release and return to the starting position.

↻ Repeat the stretch 10 times.

1. Once you have mastered the stretch lying down, you might want to progress to a seated position.

2. Sit on your chair with your legs hip-width apart and your hands on your knees. Slowly bend forward, sliding your hands down the front of your shins towards the floor, and hold for three to five seconds.

3. Slowly roll up bone by bone to return to the starting position.

Repeat 10 times.

1. Once you feel you can do the lumbar flexion from sitting, you are challenged to try it standing.

2. Stand tall with your feet hip-width apart.
   Slowly bend forward by hinging at the waist. Reach as far as you can towards your feet, and hold for three to five seconds.

3. Slowly roll back up as you imagine stacking your vertebrae.

Repeat 10 times.
You may perform any variation of this exercise multiple times a day to release tension in your back.

LUMBAR SIDE FLEXION STRETCH

INTRODUCTION

The lumbar side flexion stretch is also known as the lateral flexion stretch or side bend. It is one movement that we rarely do in our daily activities. However, if you frequent your local fitness facility for a group exercise class, chances are you will find this move included in some of the warm-up or cool-down portions of the class.

This exercise helps with lumbopelvic stability, providing pain relief to your lower back. When your lumbo-pelvic area is unstable, the force from your feet cannot travel up your spine, putting you at risk for an acute lower back injury, sharp pains in your lower back, disk degeneration, and knee issues. Picture jumping on the ground and getting the force stuck in your lower back instead of your vertebrae working to soften the blow.

The side bend motion will also help you breathe deeper because it opens the ribs.

For this exercise, sit in a chair or stand.

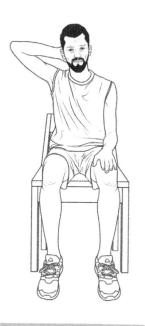
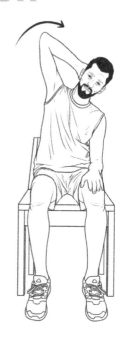

INSTRUCTIONS

1 Sitting or standing, ensure your spine is tall, and your shoulders are down and back.

2 Bring your right hand behind your head while you leave your left hand at your side.

3 Lean toward your left side to stretch the right side of your torso and hold for 10-15 seconds before releasing to return to the starting position.

↻ Repeat 10 times on each side. If you have trouble placing your right or left hand behind your head, you may put it on your lap if you are sitting or on your hip if you are standing.

SEATED ANKLE AND QUADRICEPS STRETCH

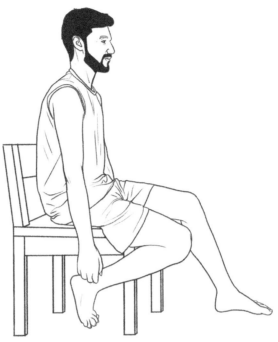

INTRODUCTION

If you are immobile or have trouble standing for long periods, try the seated ankle stretch, stretching your quads. It is important to note that a wheelchair will not work for this exercise.

INSTRUCTIONS

1. Sit on the edge of your chair, ensuring you are comfortable and not at risk of falling forward.
2. Tuck your right foot under the chair with your toes touching the floor.
3. Gently push down your foot to feel the stretch, careful not to go to the point where it causes you pain.
4. Hold from 15 to 30 seconds before switching to your left leg.

↻ Repeat five times on each side.

SEATED ANKLE STRETCH

INTRODUCTION

Ankle pain or stiffness is often the result of poor balance. Maintaining your ankles' ability is essential for daily movements such as getting up and down and walking. You will need a chair for this stretching exercise.

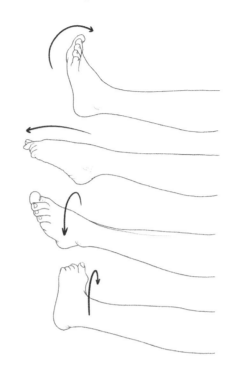

INSTRUCTIONS

1. Sit in your chair with a long spine and hands on either side of the chair.
2. Lift your right leg in front of you, just a few inches above the ground.
3. Point your toes to extend your ankle joint and hold for 10-15 seconds.
4. Bring your toes back up to flex your ankle and hold for another 10-15 seconds.
5. With your ankle still extended, push your toes to the left, leading with your baby toe and hold for 10-15 seconds.
6. Push your ankle inwards, leading with your big toe, and hold for 10-15 seconds.
7. Switch ankles.

↻ Repeat five times on each side.

CHAPTER FIVE

UPPER BODY STRETCHES

There is a very good reason why stretching and strengthening your upper back is essential.

Generally speaking, we don't always use all of the muscles in our upper backs, specifically our shoulders, in daily activities. For example, you do use both your legs to bring groceries inside your house and your arms to hold the bags, but the use of your upper back is relatively small.

Tight muscles, as you know, will not function at their optimal range.

Reaching high up to the shelves or carrying in groceries without pain will help you feel like you're living a healthier life.

In addition, maintaining strength and flexibility in your upper back allows you to have good posture.

Without a solid and flexible upper back, your muscles are more likely to feel tense, stiff, or painful, which can lead to feeling limited on things you can typically do.

ANATOMY OF YOUR UPPER BACK

Our upper backs contain muscles that begin at the skull and expand over the shoulders and down the spine to create the shape of a trapezius. The muscles' function is to help with the movement in our shoulder, neck, and scapula and to protect our upper back region. When our upper back is not maintained, the muscles become stiff and cause discomfort or pain.

A flexible body makes a big difference, especially if your neck, shoulders, and arms are tight. Upper body stretches can help you prevent tension or pain from back injuries while keeping your spine aligned. In addition, they will help your range of motion and keep it flexible.

HINTS YOU NEED TO STRETCH YOUR UPPER BACK

If you have a weak upper back, here are some of the hints that will tell you that you need to strengthen and stretch them:

- You have a hard time fully extending your arms over your head.
- You can't do a pull-up.
- You have poor posture.
- You frequently experience pain in your upper arms or shoulders.
- Your shoulders shrug during exercises.

Dynamic Upper Body Stretches

In this section, you will learn how to do dynamic upper body stretches to benefit your posture and spine so you can easily reach above your head. Remember to warm up before you get started. This could be doing some torso twists or jogging on the spot with your arms moving.

REACH AND BEND STRETCH

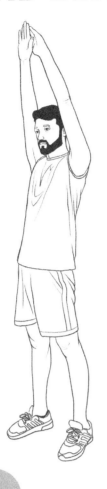
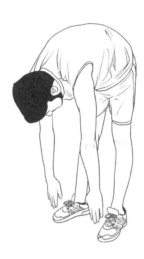

INTRODUCTION

The reach and bend stretch is a duo stretch that will help lengthen your spine while loosening tension in your lower back. You may do this exercise either seated or standing.

INSTRUCTIONS

1. Begin with your feet hip-width apart with your ankle joints under your knees.
2. Stretch both of your arms overhead and slightly arch your upper back.
3. Bend forward towards the floor and let your arms hang in front of you.

↻ Repeat 10 times.

WALL ANGEL

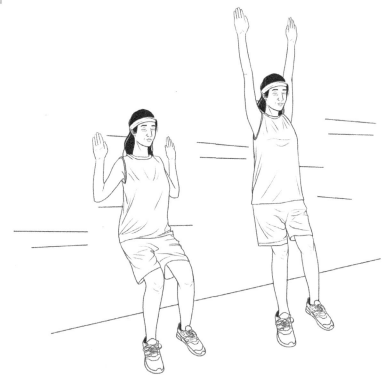

INTRODUCTION

The wall angel is an excellent stretch for your thoracic spine, requiring your upper spine to be completely flat on the wall and have your shoulder blades squeezed together.

INSTRUCTIONS

1. Sit against your wall with your legs extended out in front of you.

2. Sit tall, ensuring that your lower back is flush with the wall and your chin is slightly tucked.

3. Raise your hands to make the shape of a football goal post. Your arms, the backs of your hands, and triceps should be pressed against the wall.

4. Slowly extend your arms up overhead while maintaining contact on the wall. Pull your shoulder blades in.

5. Lower them back down in the same manner. Your back should not pull away from the wall at any point.

↻ Repeat 10-15 times.

CHEST STRETCH

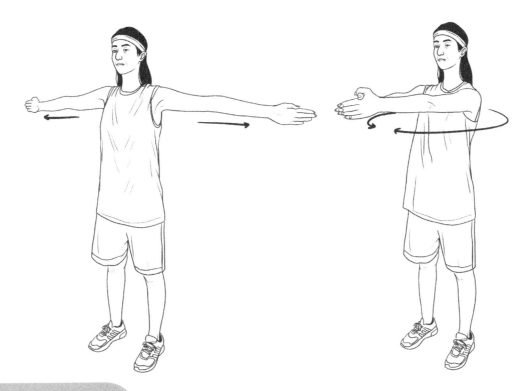

INTRODUCTION

This dynamic chest stretch will help open your pectoral muscles to allow for a better range of motion and decrease muscle tightness. In addition, if you do this stretch following an upper body workout, the stretch can provide relief to training-related shoulder pain.

INSTRUCTIONS

1. Stand or sit with your legs hip-width apart.
2. Lift your arms in front of you so they are shoulder height.
3. Continue to move your arms back as far as possible as if you are reverse clapping.

↻ Repeat 5-10 times.

NECK STRETCHES

Neck extension and flexion involve tucking your chin into your chest. Your neck's typical range of motion is between 40 and 80 degrees. The simple movement of moving your neck is something we do several times a day without thinking about it until we begin to experience pain. Some pain in your neck can be caused by sleeping the wrong way or holding your head for too long in a particular position, such as:

- Reading
- Cycling
- Long Drives
- Walking
- Sewing, drawing, writing
- Carrying heavy shoulder or duffle bags
- Sports
- Doing the same movements in your upper body

NECK EXTENSION STRETCH

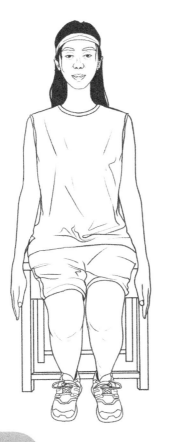
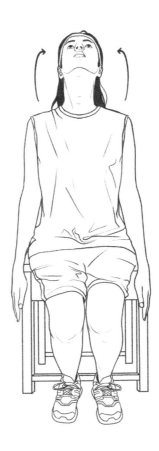

INTRODUCTION

This dynamic stretch will help loosen tight muscles, decrease spinal pressure, and relieve pain. You may do this sitting or standing.

INSTRUCTIONS

1. Sit or stand with your spine tall with your shoulders relaxed.
2. Tilt your head back as far as is comfortable with your gaze towards the ceiling.
3. Hold for two to three seconds.

Slowly bring your head back down to its normal position.

↻ Repeat three to four times for 8-10 repetitions throughout the day. One repetition is equal to three or four extensions.

SIDE REACHES

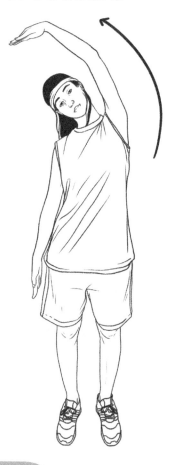
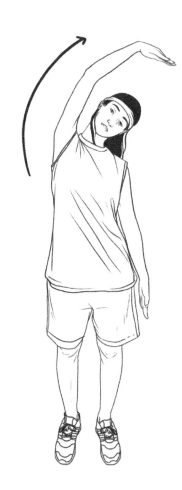

INTRODUCTION

If the side of your neck feels a little tense or achy, try doing some side reaches. The stretch targets your neck and stretches the side of your torso.

INSTRUCTIONS

1. Stand or sit tall with your core engaged.
2. Raise your right arm to the ceiling bending to the left. Your palm should be facing down toward the floor.
3. Repeat the same motion with your left arm.

↻ Alternate between your left and right arms for 10-12 repetitions.

UPPER TRAPEZIUS STRETCH

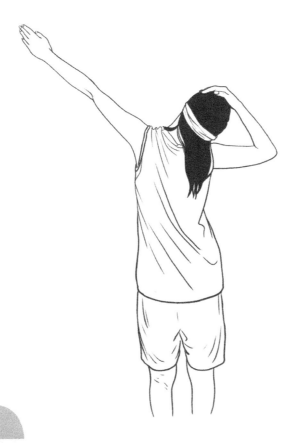

INTRODUCTION

Your trapezius muscle begins at your neck, spans the width of your shoulders, and extends to your mid-back. The trapezius muscle is in charge of the shrugging motion in your shoulders and the ability to pull your shoulders down, which is also one of the root causes of neck pain. You can do this stretch seated or standing so long as your spine is neutral and your core is engaged.

INSTRUCTIONS

1. Bring your right hand to your lower back with your elbow bent.
2. Put your left hand on top of your head.
3. Use your left hand to gently pull your head forward until you feel a stretch at the base of your neck and the upper part of your trapezius.
4. Hold for 30 seconds, and then repeat with your right hand on top of your head.

SCISSOR STRETCH

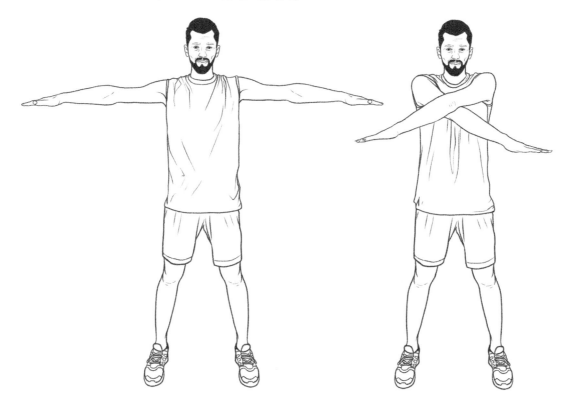

INTRODUCTION

The scissor stretch will help relieve tension in your deltoids, pectoral, upper back, biceps, and tricep muscles.

INSTRUCTIONS

1   Stand straight with a neutral spine and your shoulders down and back.

2   Extend your arms out at shoulder height.

3   Keep your elbows straight but not locked; bring both arms in front of your chest, crossing your right arm over your left arm.

4   Move your arms behind your shoulders, only going as far as is comfortable.

5   Repeat the same movement with your left arm crossing over your right.

6   Alternate back and forth, switching each time for one minute.

WRIST FLEXION

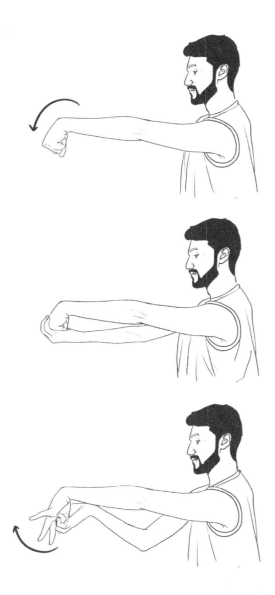

INTRODUCTION

Our wrist joint, though small, is mighty. We don't even think about it until it starts to cause discomfort or pain when trying to do things such as typing on a keyboard, using a screwdriver, or doing a downward dog-to-cobra stretch if you are a yogi. Interestingly, wrist injuries are one of the most common ones we can get because we use our wrists in almost everything we do.

This simple stretch will help keep your wrists healthy and is one you can do anytime during the day.

INSTRUCTIONS

1. Sit or stand with a neutral spine and your shoulders down and back.
2. Extend your right arm out in front of you.
3. Drop your wrist, allowing it to be weak.
4. Use your left hand to apply gentle pressure to the back of your hand, pushing your fingers towards your forearm until you feel a stretch on top of your wrist. Hold for 10 seconds, release, and then repeat.

↻ Repeat five times and then switch to your left wrist.

WRIST EXTENSION

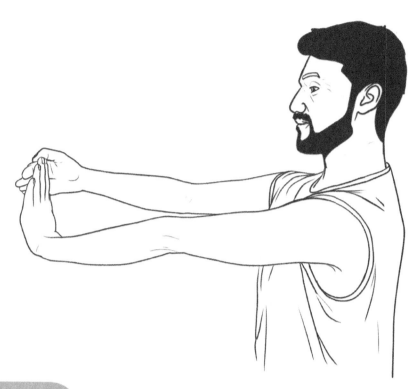

INTRODUCTION

This is the opposite movement from the flexion stretch. This time, you will feel a stretch underneath your wrists and in some of your forearms.

INSTRUCTIONS

1. Sit or stand with a neutral spine and your shoulders down and back.
2. Extend your right arm out in front of you with your palm facing down.
3. Use your left hand to bend your wrist with your fingers pointing towards the ceiling.
4. Apply gentle pressure to press your fingers toward your upper forearm. Hold for 10 seconds, release, and then repeat.

Repeat five times and then switch to your left wrist.

Static Upper Body Stretches

You can do these exercises after a workout since your arms will be warm.

UPPER BACK STRETCH

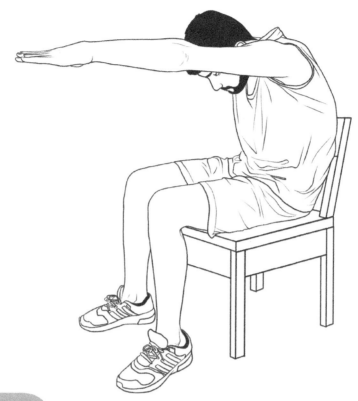

INTRODUCTION

The upper back stretch helps with the overall flexibility and reduces stiffness in your shoulder joints. It also helps with blood circulation, allowing more oxygen to reach your muscles to help them repair and reduce the risk of tension and muscle damage after a workout.

INSTRUCTIONS

1. Sit in a chair with a tall spine and your shoulders down and back.
2. Interlock your fingers and flip them, so your palms are facing out.
3. Push your palms away as you feel your shoulder blades stretch out from your spine. Hold for 10 seconds.

Repeat 5-10 times.

SHOULDER AND OVERHEAD STRETCH

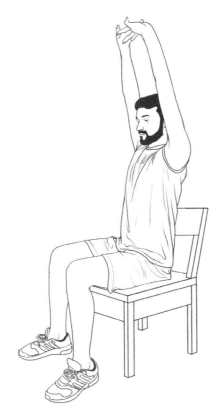

INTRODUCTION

The shoulder and overhead stretch will help you increase your shoulder's range of motion. This dual move will help you when you go to grab things from high shelves or in low cabinets.

INSTRUCTIONS

1. Sit in your chair with your spine long and shoulders down and back.
2. Bring your hands together to interlock your fingers.
3. Flip your hands to have your palms facing out.
4. Bring your hands up and above your head while keeping your fingers linked.
5. Hold for 10 seconds.
6. Release your fingers to open and lower your arms back down to the side.

↻ Repeat five times.

SHOULDER STRETCH

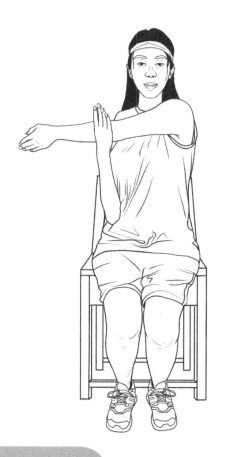
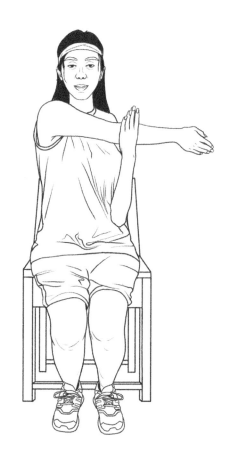

INTRODUCTION

The shoulder stretch helps your shoulder, scapula, and supporting muscles and joints to make it easier to reach across your body.

INSTRUCTIONS

1. Sit in a chair with your spine tall and shoulders down and back.
2. Bring your right arm across your body.
3. Use your left hand to hug your upper arm towards your body.
4. Hold for 15 seconds, and then release.

↻ Repeat five times before switching to your left arm.

STANDING ARMS BACKWARD STRETCH

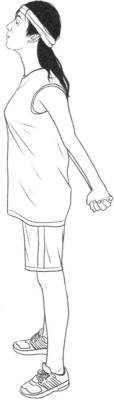

INTRODUCTION

This is probably one of the easiest and most effective chest stretches you can try. It's not only going to target your chest muscles but also your anterior shoulder and biceps.

INSTRUCTIONS

1. Stand up straight with a neutral spine. Make sure your shoulders are down and back.
2. Reach behind your back with both of your arms. Clasp your hands together.
3. Straighten your elbows and lift your chest to feel a stretch in your pectoral muscles.
4. Raise your arms a little higher to deepen the stretch if you are able.

DOOR CHEST STRETCH

INTRODUCTION

A classic stretch, but a good one! Using a doorway to stretch your chest opens your anterior shoulder and chest muscles to improve your mobility and posture. However, due to your shoulder being susceptible, be mindful that you do not overstretch your shoulders as you could injure them.

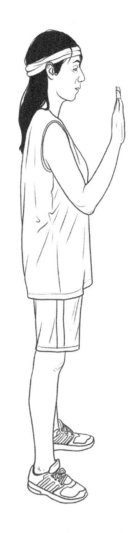
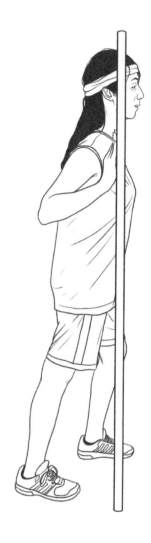

INSTRUCTIONS

1. Stand just outside of your doorway with a neutral spine.
2. Bend your elbow and bring it to shoulder height with the palm of your hand facing the front.
3. Place your elbow and upper arm against the doorway. Lean into it until you feel a stretch in your chest. Hold for 20 to 30 seconds.
4. Release and repeat on the other side.

↻ Repeat five times on each side.

NECK FLEXION STRETCH

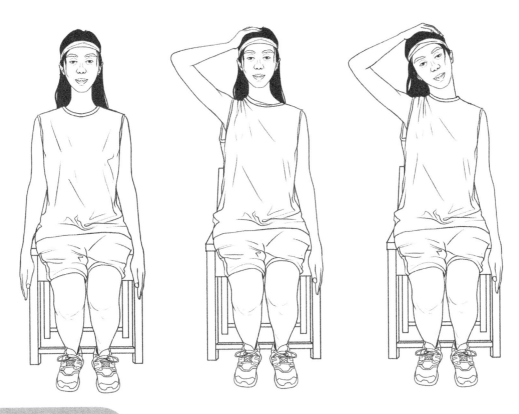

INTRODUCTION

The flexion version of the neck stretch will help reduce tightness and loosen your posterior neck muscles. You may do this exercise seated or standing.

INSTRUCTIONS

1. Sit or stand with your spine tall with your shoulders relaxed.

2. Tuck your chin as far as you can towards your chest. You should feel a slight stretch at the back of your neck. If you want to deepen the stretch, place your hands on the back of your head and apply gentle pressure.

3. Hold for between 15 and 30 seconds, and then bring your head back to its normal position.

↻ Repeat three or four times.

CHAPTER SIX
STRETCHES FOR SPECIFIC CONDITIONS

Maintaining movement when you have specific conditions, such as arthritis or sciatica, is crucial as it will help combat fatigue and joint pain and maintain or increase flexibility.

Of course, when your body is in pain, sometimes the last thing you want to do is move it. However, by not moving, you risk further tension in your body, and thus, your pain will increase.

In this chapter, the exercises have been separated between arthritis, sciatica, and nerve pain.

However, some have a dual purpose and can help with either condition.

In addition, most exercises will target lower back pain, too.

WHAT IS ARTHRITIS?

Having arthritis means that one or more of your joints are inflamed. Typical symptoms include joint pain and stiffness. This section will teach you some stretches to help alleviate arthritis pain.

SPONGE SQUEEZE

INTRODUCTION

Stress balls were designed to relieve stress and tension. However, studies have found that squeezing has other health benefits for our wrists and hands. You activate your nerves and muscles when you squeeze an object like a stress ball or a sponge that can relieve the pain you might have from arthritis. In addition, it will help strengthen your muscles, too! You can use a sponge for this or a stress ball.

Before you begin the sponge squeeze, warm up your wrists by doing some rotations for at least two minutes.

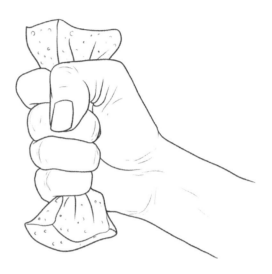

INSTRUCTIONS

1. With your sponge or stress ball in your right hand, squeeze the object to make a fist.

2. Hold for 10 seconds, and then release.

Repeat 10 times on each hand.

LOCUST POSE

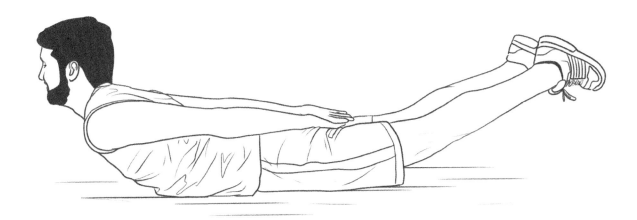

INTRODUCTION

The locust pose helps to strengthen your spine, glutes, and thighs. In addition, it will help stabilize your core and lower back while improving circulation and flexibility in your hips.

INSTRUCTIONS

1. On the floor, lie down on your stomach with your arms along your sides, palms up.
2. Inhale to slowly lift your chest, arms, and head as high as you can. Picture Superman diving down from the sky.
3. Extend your arms up and away from your torso while you squeeze your glutes, lower back, and abs.
4. Hold for 30 seconds, and then release to lower everything back down.

↻ Repeat one to two times.
If you find raising your legs off the floor is too difficult, you may leave them on the floor but ensure you activate your glutes and lower back.

Other Stretches for Arthritis

You learned some other stretches you can do in Chapters 4 and 5. Some of these are also great for relieving arthritis pain and include:

- Ankle circles

- Knee-to-chest stretch

- Butterfly stretch

- Reach and bend

- Wrist flexion and extension

WHAT ARE SCIATICA AND NERVE PAIN?

Sciatica is a condition that radiates pain along the sciatic nerve path. The sciatic nerve starts at your lower back and extends through your hips, buttocks, and down both legs. If you have sciatica, it usually only affects one side of your body.

Nerve pain, however, describes a condition in which a health condition impacts the nerves that transmits the feelings of pain to your brain. Nerve pain often differs from other pain and generally feels like a stabbing, shooting, or burning pain.

Each of these stretches can help relieve sciatica and nerve pain.

STANDING HAMSTRING STRETCH

INTRODUCTION

Use the standing hamstring stretch if you are looking to relieve pain and tightness in your hamstring caused by sciatica or arthritis. You will need an elevated surface for the stretch. A chair or an ottoman will do just fine as long as your foot is below your hips' level.

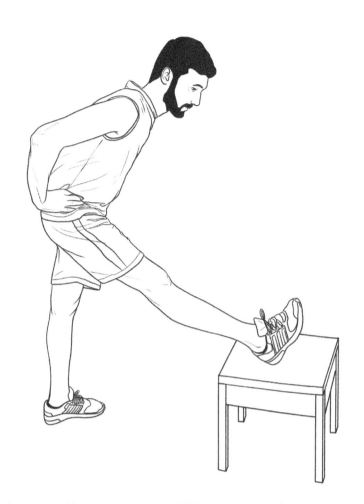

INSTRUCTIONS

1. Place your right foot on your elevated surface with your ankle flexed. Be sure to keep your supporting and working leg knee soft.

2. Hinge at your hips and reach your arms toward your foot until you feel a stretch. The further you reach, the deeper the stretch will be. However, do not bend too far where you feel pain or try to push through the pain.

3. Hold for 30 seconds.

4. Release the stretch and bring your leg down to repeat on the other side.

↻ Do one to two sets with two to three repetitions on each leg.

SITTING SPINAL TWIST

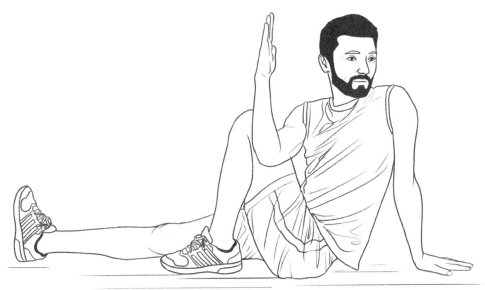

INTRODUCTION

This stretch is similar to the seated spinal twist, except it is done on the floor instead. Some sciatic pain can be triggered when your vertebrae become compressed in your spine. As we know, twisting allows your spine to reset and sends better blood and oxygen flow throughout your body for better recovery. This twist variation will also help create space in your spine so that the sciatic nerve can get the relief it needs.
This stretch can also help relieve arthritis pain.

INSTRUCTIONS

1. Sit on the floor with your legs extended out in front of you and your ankles flexed.
2. Bend and bring your right leg up, placing it over your opposite knee.
3. Bring your left elbow to the exterior side of your right knee to assist you as you gently twist your body to the right.
4. Hold for 30 seconds and then slowly untwist.
5. Repeat another two times before switching sides.

↻ Do this at least once or twice on each side, three times per set.

COBRA POSE

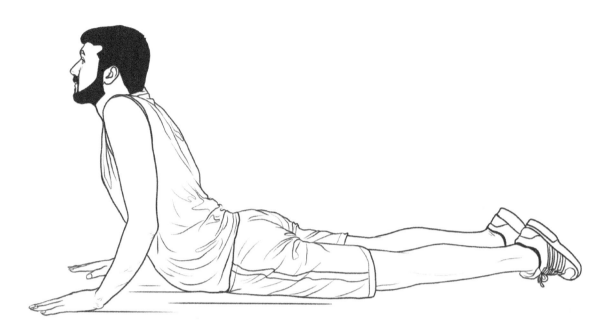

INTRODUCTION

If you suffer from sciatica, this is an excellent yoga pose to help improve the symptoms. The cobra is a backbend stretch that helps with spinal extension to bring the herniated disk forward and off the spinal nerves.

INSTRUCTIONS

1. On the floor, lie on your stomach with your palms facing down. Your hands will need to be next to your pectoral muscles.
2. Hug your elbows into your sides.
3. Have your neck in a neutral position and your eyes gazing down, inhale and lift your chest off the floor, only going as comfortable as it is for you.
4. Hold for 15 seconds and then release.

↻ Repeat five times.

CAT-COW POSE

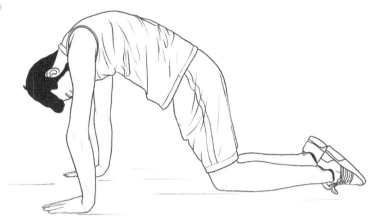

INTRODUCTION

If you deal with persistent pain in your neck, shoulders, back, and pelvis, it is likely that you are unconsciously protecting those areas, thus creating a rigid feeling in your body. The cat-cow yoga pose helps to release the tension.

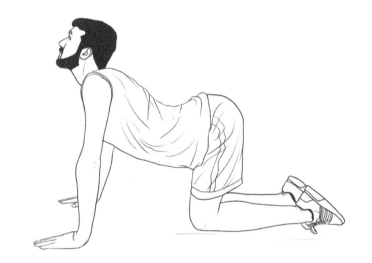

INSTRUCTIONS

1. On the floor, get on your hands and knees with your legs shoulder-width apart.
2. Inhale to tuck your pelvis in and bring your chin down to your chest to create the cat position.
3. For the cow position, exhale and lift your head and chest while pushing your tailbone to the ceiling to arch your back. Drop your stomach to the floor.
4. Repeat the movement going from cat to cow pose for one minute.

↻ If you find that having your wrists extended for a long period causes pain, try making a fist to bear your weight on it or use a weight on the ground.
You can do this yoga stretch sitting on a chair with your hands on your knees if you find it is difficult to get up and down from the floor.

BRIDGE POSE

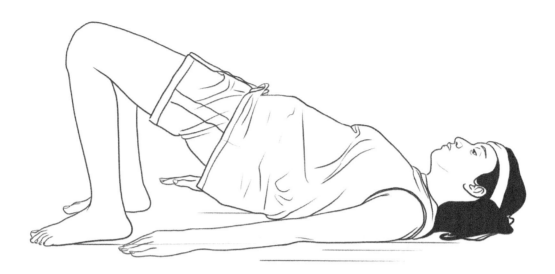

INTRODUCTION

The bridge pose helps to stretch the spine to provide relief to any pain or tension you are holding. This exercise will also help with boosting circulation while engaging your legs, glutes, and core.

INSTRUCTIONS

1. On the floor, lie on your back with your arms by your sides. Palms are facing down.
2. Slowly lift your spine from the floor while you raise your hips as high as possible and hold for 15-20 seconds.
3. Slowly lower back down.

↻ Repeat 10 times.

RECLINING PIGEON POSE

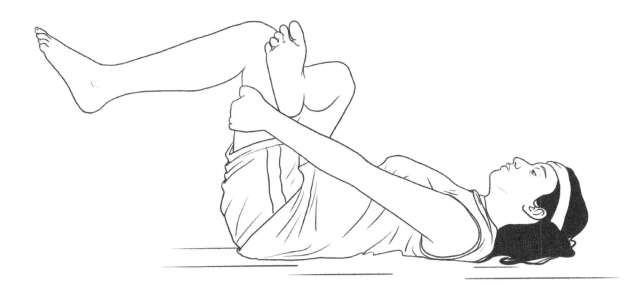

INTRODUCTION

This familiar yoga pose helps to open your hips, especially if you suffer from sciatica. In addition, this yoga pose will relieve your lower back, hamstrings, and sciatic nerve. This stretch is also good if you have arthritis.

INSTRUCTIONS

1. On your floor, lie down on your back.
2. Bend both knees, so your feet are flat on the floor.
3. Bring your right leg to a right angle and place it on your left knee.
4. Clasp your fingers behind your left leg and gently pull it towards you.
5. Hold for one minute.
6. Release and repeat with your left leg.

↻ If you find you are benefitting from the stretch, you are encouraged to stretch each leg one or two more times.

CHAPTER SEVEN

STRETCHING WITH EQUIPMENT

Stretching with equipment can add a new layer to regaining your flexibility and range of motion.

However, this does not mean you need to go out and buy a stretching machine.

Tools, such as a foam roller and a stretch band, can do the trick just fine, if not better. This chapter will introduce how to use a foam roller and a stretch band to deepen some of your stretches.

WHAT IS A FOAM ROLLER?

A foam roller is a cylinder piece of foam or ball that you can use for self-massaging purposes. With a foam roller, you use your body weight to roll over various points of your body to loosen muscle knots in the fascia and provide pressure relief to your nearby joints.

A study in 2014 found that foam rolling is an effective way to reduce stiffness and improve blood circulation to the muscles. As you age, foam rolling can:

- Help fix muscle imbalance
- Relieve muscle spasms
- Relieve fatigue following a workout by improving blood circulation
- Help with joint flexibility
- Repair muscles to boost their recovery time
- Decrease the risk of injury during any activity
- Improve movement patterns

Our fascial and myofascial makeup loses elasticity as we age; the result is that they tend to create friction as opposed to gliding across one another easily. As a result, when you experience pain is connected to your fascia when you feel like you have a knot in your muscle or that you have pulled it. As you would find with getting a massage, the foam roller will help to release the fascial tissue and increase circulation in the area through the pressure of the foam roller.

Thus, the foam roller is worth trying if you want to loosen your tight muscles, relieve aches and pains, and promote overall relaxation. In addition, it can help align your body so you can move easily.

You may also want to use a menthol massage gel or essential oil before or after your foam rolling session. Once you conclude foam rolling, a hot shower or bath is recommended to apply heat and soothe the areas you worked on.

Types of Foam Rollers

Here are the different types of foam rollers you can find in a fitness store or online:

- Soft foam rollers are low density and recommended for those newer to foam rolling or if you have sensitivities.
- Firm foam rollers are high density and apply more pressure on your body.
- Textured foam rollers have grids, knobs, or ridges to help target your muscles more deeply.
- Travel foam rollers are suitable for your arms or calves and are easier to travel to the gym with.
- Vibrating foam rollers have a different setting that will help loosen tight or tense muscles and release fascial knots. This type of foam roller can help with improving flexibility and circulation.
- Heated or cool foam rollers can help promote muscle relaxation and help with discomfort.
- Foam roller balls are good for targeting specific areas such as feet.
- Foam rolling sticks apply direct pressure on the areas causing pain.

Do's and Don'ts of Foam Rolling

1. Do research on which foam roller is best for you. Each one has a different length, diameter, and density. Most rollers are between 12 and 36 inches. However, the rule of thumb you should follow is that if you are newer to foam rolling or have sensitivities, softer is better.
2. Start with 10 minutes at a time and then slowly progress as you get used to foam

1. rolling. Make sure you are easing into the rolling movement by going in different directions, such as front to back and side to side.

2. Do expect a little bit of pain. It's normal as foam rolling applies firm pressure to a tight or sore muscle. Foam rolling is not meant to hurt; if it hurts you, back off on the pressure.

3. Never roll directly on your joints, bones, or iliotibial band. Repeated rolling on your joints or bones can result in inflammation. Your iliotibial band is a large tendon that runs on the exterior of your thigh between your hip and knee. Since your iliotibial band is not a muscle, you will only feel nerve pain that runs through it and causes inflammation. If you have issues with the iliotibial band, your best option is to roll the muscles surrounding it, such as your glutes, hamstrings, and quads. We'll get into that during the exercise section of the chapter.

4. Do seek the advice of a professional if you have neck pain. Your neck is one of the most sensitive areas in your body and is too sensitive for foam rolling. If you foam roll your neck, you could cause severe injury.

5. Don't roll your lower back because it can cause your spine to contract.

6. Do roll slowly, moving one inch per second.

7. Do roll over your trigger points 5-10 times, spending no more than 30 seconds on your tender spots.

8. Don't roll to the point that you have excessive soreness.

9. Don't foam roll if you have injuries in specific areas.

10. Do wait 24 to 48 hours between rolling sessions.

Make sure you are warmed up before you begin to foam roll.

PECTORALS AND CHEST

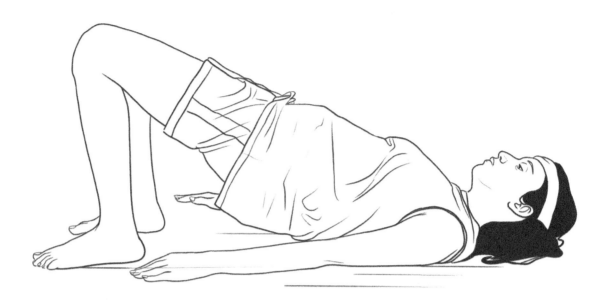

INTRODUCTION

Using a foam roller on your pectorals and chest will help to reduce tightness in the chest muscles and improve your shoulders' mobility. A shorter foam roller is best for this exercise.

INSTRUCTIONS

1. Lie face down on your yoga mat or floor and place the foam roller parallel to your body under your right pectoral muscle, close to your shoulder.
2. Bend your right arm 90 degrees. You may leave your left arm where it's comfortable for you so long as your head remains lifted off the ground.
3. Lean into the foam roller as you roll toward and away from your elbow, inch by inch. If you hit a tender spot, pause for a moment and breathe into it. Continue for 90 seconds to two minutes.Repeat on the other side.

LATISSIMUS DORSI

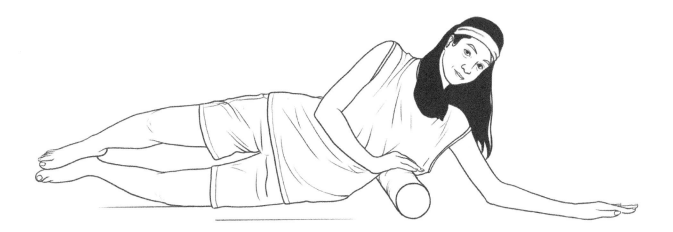

INTRODUCTION

Using a foam roller on your latissimus dorsi, you can find that the muscle tension below your underarms can be alleviated. In addition, stretching can help improve your posture and mobility in your upper body.

INSTRUCTIONS

1. Lie on your right side.
2. Put the foam roller under your right shoulder.
3. Bend your right leg slightly and bring your left leg up with your foot planted on the floor in front of your right leg.
4. Starting just below your armpit, roll down toward your mid-back. If you feel any pressure points, pause for a moment.
5. Continue for 60 to 90 seconds, and then switch sides.

↻ Repeat three times on the right and left.

UPPER BACK

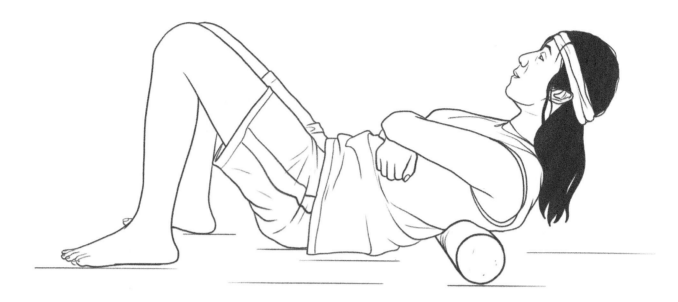

INTRODUCTION

A foam roller along your spine can help align and release muscle knots, tension, and tightness. In addition, this exercise can help improve your posture, especially if you sit for extended periods. You will need a longer foam roller for this stretch.

INSTRUCTIONS

1. On the floor, lie on the roller parallel to your spine, ensuring your head and tailbone are supported.
2. Bend your knees up to place your feet flat on the floor.
3. Spread your arms wide with your palms facing the ceiling and feel your shoulder blades squeeze against the roller.
4. Breathe and relax into the position and hold for two to three minutes.

↻ Repeat two or three more times as needed.

SPINAL ALIGNMENT

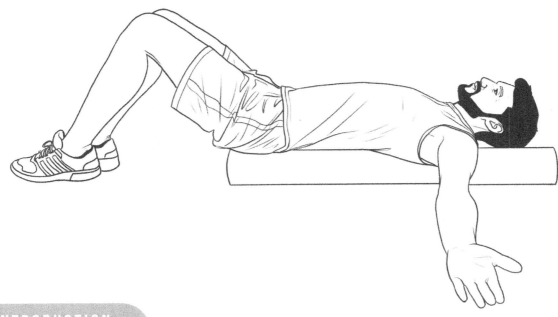

INTRODUCTION

Our middle back muscles are some of the hardest muscles to reach. Thankfully with a foam roller, it makes the muscles reachable. If you have back issues, be careful or avoid this stretch.

INSTRUCTIONS

1. Sit on the floor with your knees bent to the ceiling.
2. Bring your foam roller behind you and lean back, putting your shoulder blades on top of the roller to position your middle back.
3. Join your fingers behind your head. You can also cross your arms with your hands on opposite shoulders.
4. While holding your head, look up as you slowly lower your upper back into the roller, feeling the tension release from your mid-back. Hold for one to two minutes, then slowly sit back to a seated position.

↻ Try gently rolling your back to massage the tender areas if you like.

LOWER BACK

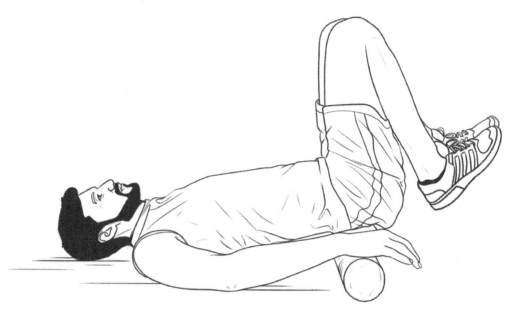

INTRODUCTION

You can use a foam roller to release tension in your lower back. However, be sure not to put too much pressure or roll your lower back, as you will risk your spine contracting and causing a spasm.

INSTRUCTIONS

1. On the floor, bring your foam roller so that it is horizontal to your lower back.
2. Put your feet flat on the floor with your knees bent towards the ceiling.
3. Bring your knees to your chest, holding your shins with your hands. You may also place your hands on your hamstrings behind your knees if that is more comfortable.
4. Gently move your legs to the right side to raise the left side of your lower back from the foam roller, hold for five seconds, and then gently rock to the other side.
5. Continue to gently rock side to side for one minute.

↻ Repeat two to three times.

CORE

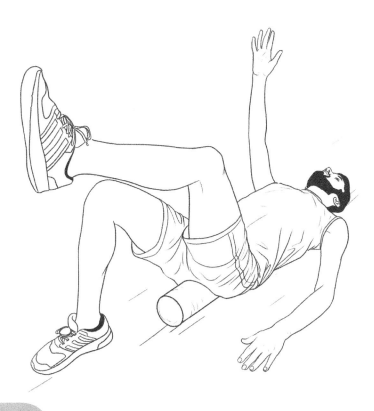

INTRODUCTION

A foam roller can help increase your core's strength to support posture, stability, and alignment further. You will need a longer foam roller for this exercise.

INSTRUCTIONS

1. On the floor, lie on the roller parallel to your spine, ensuring your head and tailbone are supported.

2. Have your knees bent and feet firmly pressed on the floor with your arms alongside your body.

3. As you push your lower back into the foam roller, engage your core muscles and simultaneously lift your left knee and right hand toward the ceiling.

4. Lower your back to the starting position and repeat with the opposite side to complete one repetition.

↻ Repeat 12-16 times for one to three sets.

GLUTEUS MAXIMUS

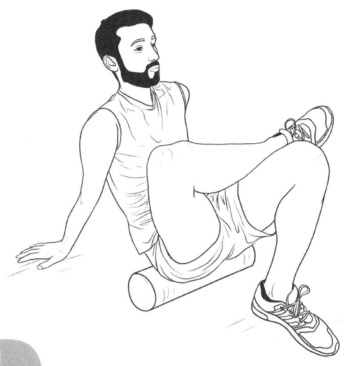

INTRODUCTION

The foam roller can help your glutes by loosening stiff legs and supporting your lower back. A long foam roller is best for this exercise.

INSTRUCTIONS

1. On the floor, sit on the foam roller and put your hands behind your hips for support.
2. Bring your knees up to a point to the ceiling and put your feet flat on the floor.
3. Cross your right ankle over your left knee.
4. Bring your left hand to your right ankle or thigh and lean onto the right to stretch your glutes.
5. Roll from side to side to target pressure points, holding for 30 seconds. Repeat on the left side.

Repeat three times on each leg.

QUADRICEPS

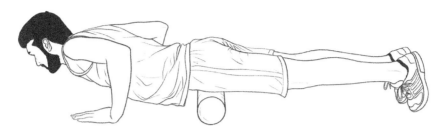

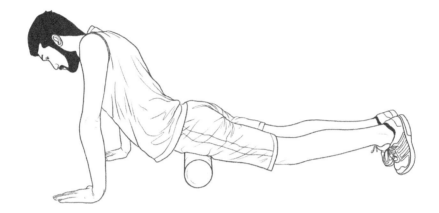

INTRODUCTION

If you want to increase flexibility in your quads, try rolling them out with this exercise.

INSTRUCTIONS

1. Lie down on the floor and place the foam roller under your quad. It might be more comfortable to open your left hip and have the inside of your left knee on the floor.

2. Begin with the lower part of your quad, rolling up and down.

3. Move to the upper part of your quad, repeating the same motion being careful not to roll onto your hip bones.

↻ If you hit any pressure points, flex your ankle and toes and hold for a moment. Continue for 90 seconds to two minutes.

CALVES

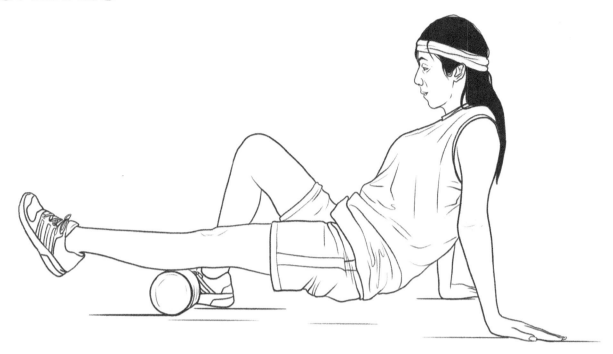

INTRODUCTION

Foam rolling can help your calves loosen up following exercise.

INSTRUCTIONS

1. Sit on the floor with your left knee bent with the foam roller under your right calf. Put your hands on either side of your knee for stability.

2. Using your hands, lift your hips off the floor as you roll the bottom half of your half forward and backward.

3. Repeat on the upper calf.

↻ Ensure you stop on tender areas and gently rotate your leg side to side in the upper and lower parts of your calf muscle.

Switch between the upper and lower parts for 90 seconds to two minutes, then switch legs.

FEET

INTRODUCTION

Foam rolling your feet can help relieve tired and achy feet. It can also help your body move better as the release can increase flexibility in the hamstrings and lower back. Any size foam roller can work for this, or a foam rolling ball would also suffice.

Use a chair or wall for stability for support if needed. Otherwise, both of your hands can remain on your hips.

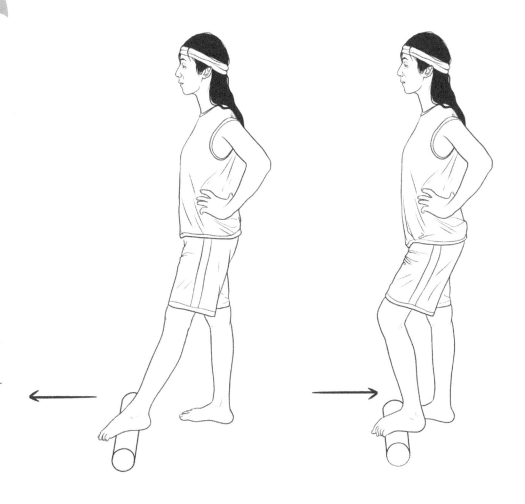

INSTRUCTIONS

1. Stand with the foam roller or ball under your right foot.
2. Roll through your feet and arches forward, backward, and laterally over pressure points.
3. Continue for 90 seconds to two minutes.

RESISTANCE STRETCHING

Resistance stretching is a way to improve and expand your range of motion. It can also help you restore your fascia to its normal length. However, since most of the joints in our body are synovial joints, movement can feel strained, problematic, or painful when the tissue surrounding the joint becomes tight. It is estimated that about 45% of the tightness in our bodies results from our joint capsules becoming tight, from compression and stiffness due to sitting or poor sleeping patterns. Resistance bands will pull on the joint you are trying to stretch to create more space between the joints.

Other benefits of using a resistance band include:

- Improved balance to reduce the risk of falls

- Improved posture

- Reduced risk of injury

- Increased bone density

- Enhanced ability to perform everyday tasks

- Improved muscle tone and strength

Type of Bands

The following are the commonly used resistance bands for stretching or training:

- Tube bands with handles look a bit like a jump rope. Their resistance ranges between 10 and 50 pounds.
- Loop bands are commonly used for various weight resistances to add extra tension or assist in exercises such as pull-ups. These bands range between five and 175 pounds.

- Therapy bands longer than a tube or loop band offer less resistance. These bands are excellent if you are recovering from an injury or surgery as they can stretch up to seven feet. This type of band is one of the best to start with if you are newer to using resistance bands for stretching. Therapy bands' resistance ranges from three to 10 pounds.
- Mini bands are a more petite version of a loop band and come in rubber or fabric. These are primarily used in lower body exercises. Their resistance ranges between five and 50 pounds.

A note regarding resistance weights: The resistance weight noted for each type of band reflects the amount of weight it would take for the resistance band to reach its maximum strength. It is not reflective of an actual weight amount.

CHEST BAND PULL

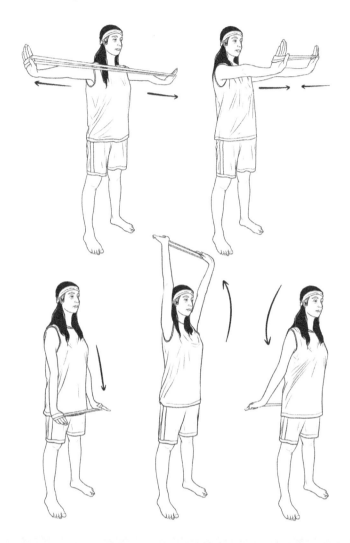

Using a resistance band for your chest muscles will help to open your chest while working your shoulders, rhomboids, biceps, lats, and pectoral muscles.

INSTRUCTIONS

1. Stand with your feet hip-width apart.
2. Grasp your band on each end and hold it out in front of you with your arms shoulder-width apart and palms facing up.
3. Extend your arms wide as you pull the band towards your chest, contracting your shoulder blades.

CHEST OPENER

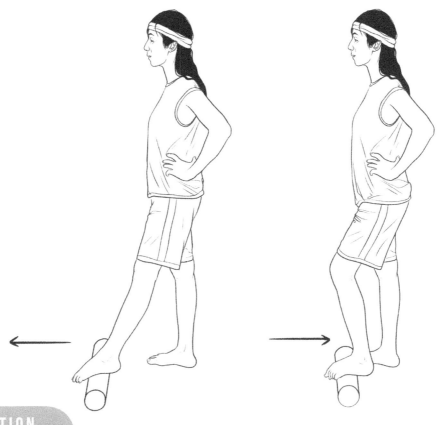

INTRODUCTION

This stretch targets your shoulders and chest to help with your range of motion and release any pectoral tension.

INSTRUCTIONS

1. Stand with your feet hip-width apart.
2. Hold each end of the band out in front of you with your palms down.
3. Bring the band up and over your head, extending your arms as far back behind you as you can.
4. Hold for five seconds
5. Bring your band back out in front of you.

↻ Repeat 5-10 times in total.

KNEELING SHOULDER STRETCH

INTRODUCTION

The kneeling shoulder stretch will help your upper back release tension. A loop band is the best option for this exercise.

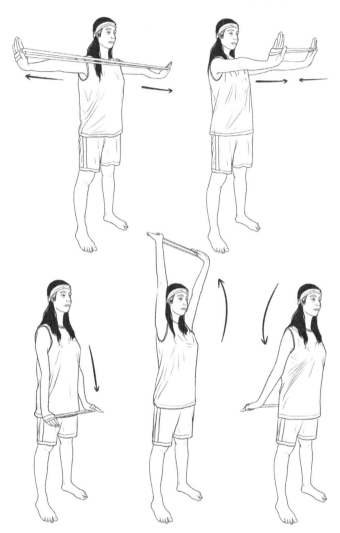

INSTRUCTIONS

1. Kneel on your knees with your ankle in the loop of the band.

2. With your hands, grab the band with your palms facing forward. Be sure not to twist the band. It should remain one open loop from your hands down to your ankle.

3. Stretch both hands over your head and push your chest out to create a slight arch in your back. The more you push your chest out and arch your upper back, the deeper the stretch will be.

4. Hold for 15 seconds and release.

↻ Repeat up to five times.

UPPER BACK STRETCH

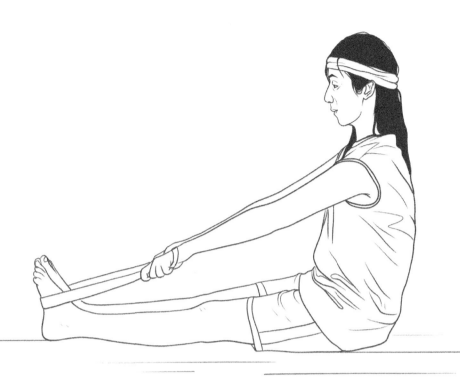

INTRODUCTION

This is a different variation to stretch out your lower back. The therapy resistance band is recommended; however, a loop band will suffice.

INSTRUCTIONS

1. Sit on the floor with your legs extended in front of you.
2. Put your resistance band around the arches of your feet.
3. Exhale, round your back away from your toes, and hold for 30 seconds.

HAMSTRING STRETCH

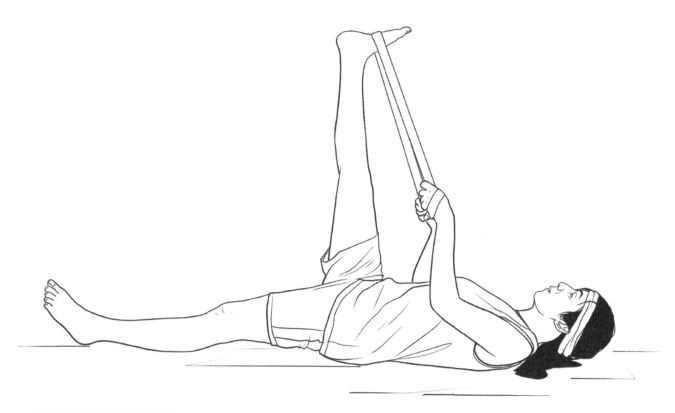

INTRODUCTION

This is a different way to stretch your hamstring while working on the range of motion in your hip flexor. The stretch can also help stretch your calves.

INSTRUCTIONS

1. Lie down on your back and loop your resistance band around the arch of your right foot. You may leave your left leg bent slightly beside you or straight.

2. Make sure your lower back remains flush to the floor or yoga mat, lift your right leg and use the resistance band to pull it closer to you. Don't worry about if your leg bends as you pull it toward you.

3. Hold for 10 seconds and repeat three times on each leg.

CHAPTER EIGHT

POST-WORKOUT STRETCHES

Have you ever noticed how your muscles ache after a vigorous workout?

This is because the body produces lactic acid, which makes your muscles feel exhausted and sore.

Stretching helps to eliminate the lactic acid buildup while relaxing your muscles.

You also want to bring your blood flow to the muscles you worked to prevent stiffness and lessen the recovery time.

WHAT IS RECOVERY TIME?

During the recovery time, most muscle and strength are usually built due to protein synthesis increasing by about 50%.

Recovery is an essential part of workouts because it allows you to:

- Rebuild muscle fibers
- Restore fluid
- Remove metabolic waste (the lactic acid buildup)

During your recovery, this is a great moment to go for a walk or maybe do a light stationary bicycle ride. But, you can do simply nothing at all and rest.

POST-WORKOUT STRETCHES

The various stretching exercises in previous chapters can be used after your workouts. These are just a few more you can use following a workout, some of which will target specific areas such as your legs and arms. Remember to be warmed up before attempting any stretches to reduce the risk of injury.

SEATED HAMSTRING STRETCH

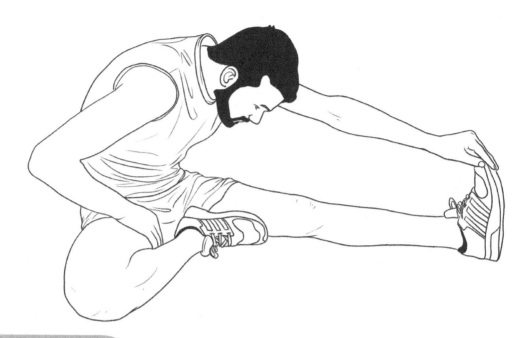

INTRODUCTION

The hamstring stretch will target your lower back and legs. This stretch is vital for seniors to help loosen stiffness and help maintain mobility in your back and legs. In addition, this variation can be helpful if you have sciatica or nerve pain.

You will need to sit on the floor for the hamstring stretch. You have a couple of options for the seated position:

- You can sit with your legs out in a V-shape.
- You can extend one leg out and bend the other knee to place your foot into your inner thigh.

Make sure not to over-extend your legs to the point that it causes discomfort.

INSTRUCTIONS

1. Lean forward towards your right leg, breathe, and reach for your ankle, thigh, or knee.
2. Hold for 20 to 30 seconds before sitting back up.

SIDE STRETCH

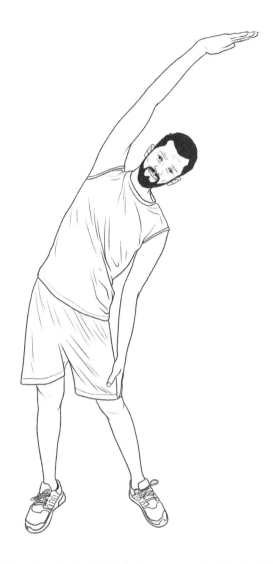

INTRODUCTION

The side stretch helps to lengthen and stretch your intercostal muscles. This stretch is beneficial following a core-focused workout.

INSTRUCTIONS

1. Standing or sitting, bring your right arm over your head and bend to the left to feel a stretch on your right side.
2. Hold the stretch for 15 seconds, and then switch sides.

↻ Repeat 10 times on both sides.

LYING PECTORAL STRETCH

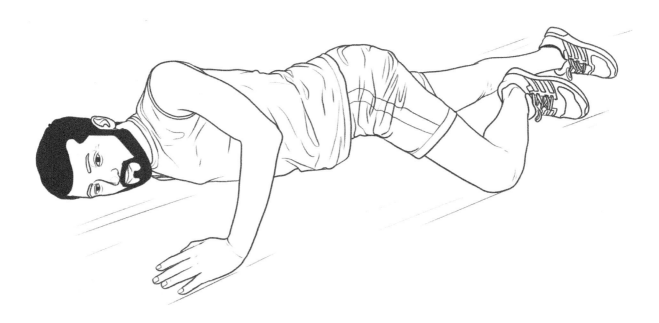

INTRODUCTION

The lying pectoral stretch allows you to target and stretch both shoulders individually.

INSTRUCTIONS

1. Lie on your stomach and place your arms out in a "T" shape.
2. As you roll to your right side, use your left hand to push off the ground as you bend your left knee for balance.
3. You will feel a stretch in your pectoral muscles on the right side. Be sure only to go as far as is comfortable. Hold for 30 seconds and then return to the starting "T" position.

↻ Repeat on the other side. Complete five repetitions on each side.

TRICEPS STRETCH

INTRODUCTION

The triceps stretch will help relieve pain and discomfort in your upper arms. In addition, performing the stretch will help lengthen your muscles and improve your flexibility while supporting your overall range of motion.

Don't do this stretch if it causes you severe pain or discomfort.

This stretch can be done seated or standing.

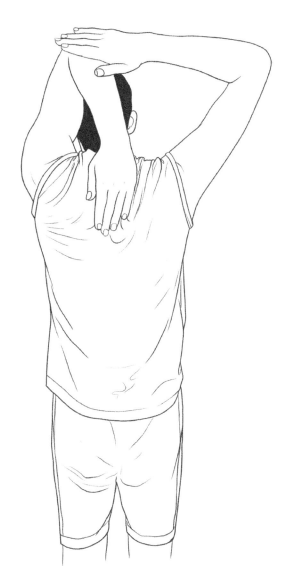

INSTRUCTIONS

1. Position your legs hip-width apart.
2. Bring both of your arms above your head.
3. Bend your right elbow to place the hand behind your head.
4. Using your left arm, gently pull your right elbow towards the middle of your back until your upper arm feels a stretch. Hold for 15 to 30 seconds and then release.
5. Repeat on the other side.

Do a total of five repetitions for each arm.

CHILD'S POSE

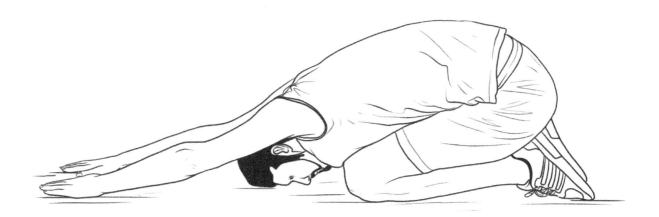

INTRODUCTION

The child's pose is one of the best stretches you can do after a workout as it helps decompress your spine, hips, core, and ankle while relieving back and neck tension. It's also excellent for calming your mind and body.

INSTRUCTIONS

1. Kneel on your knees on the floor or on a yoga mat. Have your knees a bit wider than your hips or as comfortable as it is for you.
2. Shift your buttocks towards your feet.
3. Bend forward to bring your belly between your thighs and place your forehead on the floor. Be sure to relax your shoulders, jaw, and eyes. Use a cushion if you find putting your forehead on the floor uncomfortable. Your arms can be above your head with your palms on the floor or alongside your torso and legs.

Hold for five minutes, breathing into the stretch.

CHAPTER NINE

WEEKLY WORKOUT PLANNER

This section contains various workout planners you can follow and implement into your daily routine. Make sure your body is warm before you proceed with the stretches to prevent an injury or straining your muscles.
When choosing to follow one of the five workout plans, choose one that is going to cater to what your body needs. For example, if you worked out your legs, you might want to choose some stretches exercises that will target that area.

WORKOUT PLANS INCLUDED

The five workout plans include:

- A total body plan that targets various parts of your body throughout the week

- Arthritis and sciatica

- Equipment focused stretches

- Morning and night routines

- Stretches you can do in 10 minutes

Total Body

In this workout plan, it is designed to target different areas per day.

Monday

Targeted area: upper body and back

- 5-10 windmills

- 10 to 20 shoulder rolls in both directions

- 10 reach and bends

- 10-15 wall angels

- 5-10 chest stretches

Tuesday

Targeted area: hips

- 10-15 leg swings on both sides

- 10 ankle circles per leg in both directions

- 10 knee-to-chest, holding for 20 to 30 seconds

- Five hip flexors on each leg, holding for 10-15 seconds

- Two butterfly stretches, holding 15 seconds each

Wednesday

Targeted area: lower back and legs

- Five waist loosening for two minutes each repetition
- 5-10 torso twists for two minutes each repetition
- 10 lumbar flexion stretches, holding for 10-15 seconds each time
- 10 lumbar extension stretches, holding for 10-15 seconds each time
- Five seated ankle and quadriceps stretches, holding for 15 to 30 seconds each time
- Child's pose for five minutes

Thursday

Targeted area: neck

- Four neck extension stretch for eight to 10 repetitions
- Four neck flexion stretch for eight to 10 repetitions
- 10 to 12 side reaches on each side
- Upper trapezius stretch, 30 seconds once per side

Friday

Targeted area: upper and lower back

- 10 to 20 shoulder blade squeezes
- 10 to 20 shoulder rolls
- 10 reach and bends
- 5-10 upper back stretch five times
- Five door chest stretch five times
- Child's pose for five minutes

Saturday

Targeted area: arms

- Scissor stretch for one minute

- 10 reach and bends
- Wrist flexion five times for 10 seconds each
- Wrist extension fie times for 10 seconds each
- Five lying pectoral stretch, holding 30 seconds each
- Five triceps stretch on each arm, holding for 15 to 30 seconds

Sunday

Targeted area: legs

- Walking lunges, 10 steps four times
- Walking knee hugs for 30 seconds
- Five seated ankle stretches on each leg, holding for 10-15 seconds
- Five seated ankle and quadriceps stretches, holding for 15 to 30 seconds
- Two to three seated hamstring stretches on each leg, holding for 30 seconds

SPECIFIED CONDITIONS

This workout plan has been divided between arthritis and sciatica. It is recommended that you only do each of these no more than three times a week.

Arthritis

Arms and Wrists

- 10 sponge squeeze, holding 10 seconds per squeeze
- Five wrist flexion, holding for 10 seconds each time
- Five wrist extension, holding for 10 seconds each time

Upper Back and Chest

- 10 reach and bend
- 10-15 back extensions, holding for 5-10 seconds

- 10 knee-to-chest, holding for 30 seconds per leg

- Cat-cow for one minute, three times

- Three sitting spinal twists, one to two times in each direction

Legs

- Locust poses, 30 seconds one to two times

- Butterfly stretches, 15 seconds twice

- 10 ankle circles per leg in both directions

- Two to three standing hamstrings for two repetitions

Sciatica

- Cobra pose, five times holding for 15 seconds

- Cat-cow for one minute, three times

- Bridge pose, 10 times holding for 15 to 20 seconds

- One or two reclining pigeon poses, holding for one minute per leg

- Two to three standing hamstrings for two repetitions

- Three sitting spinal twist, one to two times in each direction

Stretch Equipment Plan

As you were introduced to two different ways to utilize equipment in your stretches in Chapter 7, this workout plan has been split between foam rolling and resistance bands. Remember that if you are foam rolling to give yourself at least 24 to 48 hours in between before you foam roll again.

Foam Roller Stretches

Target: upper arms and back

- Pectoral and chest, once on each side

- Latissimus dorsi, three times each side

- Upper back two to three times, holding the stretch for two to three minutes

- One to two minutes of spinal alignment

- Lower back for one minute, going side to side two to three times

Target: core and legs

- Core, 12-16 times for one to three sets

- Gluteus maximus for 30 seconds, three times on each leg

- Quadriceps, do each leg twice for 90 seconds to two minutes

- Calves, do each leg for 90 seconds to two minutes

- Feet, do each foot twice for 90 second to two minutes

Resistance Band Stretches

- 10-15 chest band pulls

- 5-10 chest band openers

- Five kneeling shoulder stretches, holding for 15 seconds each

- Five upper back stretches, holding for 30 seconds

- Hamstring stretches three times per leg, holding for 10 seconds

Morning and Night Routines

For these routines, be sure to warm up before you start. This could be a good time to go for a morning or evening walk!

Morning

- 5-10 torso twists for two minutes each repetition

- 10 reach and bends

- 10-15 wall angels

- Four neck extension stretches for eight to 10 repetitions

- Cobra poses, five times holding for 15 seconds

- Three sitting spinal twists, one to two times in each direction
- Five hip flexors on each leg, holding for 10-15 seconds
- Two butterfly stretches, holding 15 seconds each
- One or two reclining pigeon poses, holding for one minute per leg
- Child's poses for five minutes

10-Minute Stretches

Here are two quick 10-minute stretches you can implement into your day following a brisk walk or light aerobic activity.

10-Minute Plan A

- Five waist loosening for two minutes for each repetition
- Scissor stretches for one minute
- Cat-cows for two minutes
- Child's poses for five minutes

10-Minute Plan B

- Bridge pose for two minutes
- Sponge squeeze for two minutes
- Cobra pose, four times for 15 seconds each
- Child's pose for five minutes

CONCLUSION

One of the most noticeable things we feel as we age is our flexibility and mobility starting to decrease. In addition, we begin to experience pains or aches in our legs, back, or arms when we engage in daily activities such as walking or more vigorous routines like playing tennis. The reality is that we can't stop aging, but we can do things to promote healthy aging and prevent the pain, aches, and strains that come with it.

This doesn't mean you need to stop doing what you are doing just because you ache. For example, if you love going for long hikes, you still can and are encouraged to do so. This book has given you the tools you can utilize in your day to remain flexible and mobile.

A New Flexible You

Throughout the chapters, you have learned why it is essential to be stretching. Stretching after a workout not only helps release tension and build-up of lactic acid in our muscles, but it also provides other benefits such as:

- Injury prevention
- Mindfulness
- Stress release

In addition, stretching helps you prepare for the next day's activities and to do them with less pain. The long-term effects can give you an improved posture, balance, flexibility, range of motion, body awareness, and, in some cases, weight loss and control. These are all surface-level benefits but are essential to consider.

This book has also touched on chronic conditions. Chronic conditions do not mean skipping out on a workout or stretching; it's the opposite. When we don't move, we give our muscles reasons to become tighter and therefore cause more pain or discomfort.

Although there has been much debate on stretching, such as the type of stretching and when to do it, one thing that should be made clear is that warming up is important. A brisk walk around the block will do just fine, or you can try some jumping jacks or march on the spot. So long as you get your body temperature warm, you can do a little bit of light stretching before and after; however, the static portion of stretching is always recommended to perform at the end of a workout. You should also have taken from this book how our bodies are affected by inactivity. Within various chapters, you were given different exercises to target your lower and upper body, how to manage and stretch conditions such as arthritis and sciatica, and equipment you can utilize to deepen the stretches. Listening to your body will help you determine the stretches and equipment that are best for you so you can get the most out of the stretch and help alleviate any chronic pain. The workout plans also include different targeted areas to address those pain points.

I hope that everything provided in this book ignites you to work on your flexibility so that you can live a pain-free life and continue to engage in activities that you love.

Take the exercises in this book and apply them, as I am sure they will provide you with all the benefits you are looking for.

Thank You!

This is a quick message of thanks that you picked my book from dozens of other books available for you to purchase.

Thank you for getting this and reading this all the way to the end.

Before you go, I'd like to ask a minute of your time to leave me a review on Amazon. As an indie author, every review (or star rating) matters as it helps our books become more visible on the platform thus in turn helps us reach and help more people.

Here are the links for your convenience:

Leave a review in:

US   **UK**   **CA**

GLOSSARY

Cartilage: an elastic tissue that provides cushioning between the bones.

Fascia: connective tissue that links the body's structures, such as muscles.

Iliotibial band: also known as an "IT" band, this thick fibrous tissue extends along the outside of your thigh.

Intercostal muscles: the muscles located between your rib cage.

Latissimus dorsi: a large muscle that makes up most of the upper back.

Mitochondria: a weight loss cell found in the muscles.

Oblique: the flat thin muscles between the middle and outer layers of the lateral walls of the abdomen.

Osteoporosis: a condition where bone mass decreases and causes fragility within the bone spaces.

Pectoral: the skeletal muscles that connect the chest to the upper arms.

Proprioceptive neuromuscular facilitation: a stretching technique to improve muscle elasticity.

REFERENCES

9 Easy Resistance Band Exercises for Seniors | Camino Retirement Apartments. (n.d.). Camino Retirement Apartments. https://caminoretirement. com/2018/08/28/9-easy-resistance-band-exercises-for-seniors/

9 Stretching Exercises for Seniors. (2021, May 25). Iora Primary Care. https:// ioraprimarycare.com/blog/stretching-exercises-for-seniors/

12 Minute Athlete. (2018, March 5). 6 Resistance Band Stretches for Increased Flexibility. Www.youtube.com. https://www.youtube.com/watch?v=zpTdBAl622o

Bataineh, A. (2021, December 15). Why we lose flexibility with age and what to do about it. Www.span.health. https://www.span.health/blog/why-we-lose-flexibility-with-age-and-what-to-do-about-it

Benefits of Stretching after Workouts - Diversified Integrated Sports Clinic. (2016, May 18). Diversified Integrated Sports Clinic. https://www.disc-me.com/benefits-of-stretching-after-workouts/

Blanchard, J. (2022, February 2). Stretching and Chronic Pain | Twin Cities Pain Clinic. Twin Cities Pain Clinic. https://twincitiespainclinic.com/stretching-and-chronic-pain/

Bramble, L.-A. (2021, April 19). Static vs. Dynamic Stretching: What Are They and Which Should You Do? Hospital for Special Surgery. https://www.hss.edu/article_static_dynamic_stretching.asp

Bubnis, D. (2019, July 24). Yoga for Sciatica Pain: 10 Exercises for Relief, Plus Poses to Avoid. Healthline. https://www.healthline.com/health/yoga-for-sciatica

Cain, L. (n.d.). The Dos and Don'ts of Foam Rolling - A Beginner's Guide to SMR. HFE. Retrieved September 5, 2022, from https://www.hfe.co.uk/blog/the-dos-and-donts-of-foam-rolling

Capritto, A. (2020, December 27). The Only 9 Stretches You Need to Relieve Tension in Your Neck. Verywell Fit. https://www.verywellfit.com/stretches-to-relieve-tension-in-your-neck-5084775

Capritto, A. (2021, March 9). How to do Thoracic Extensions: Techniques, Benefits, Variations. Verywell Fit. https://www.verywellfit.com/thoracic-extensions-techniques-benefits-variations-5090734

Chertoff, J. (2019, June 24). Walking Lunges: How-To, Variations, Benefits, Safety, and More. Healthline. https://www.healthline.com/health/exercise-fitness/walking-lunges

Clarke, D. (2014, June 17). Physiotherapy & Sports Injury Clinics | The Physio Company. Physiotherapy & Sports Injury Clinics | the Physio Company. https://www.thephysiocompany.com/blog/stop-slouching-postural-dysfunction-symptoms-causes-and-treatment-of-bad-posture

Cronkleton, E. (2019a, May 23). Tricep Stretches: 4 Stretches, Benefits, and More. Healthline. https://www.healthline.com/health/exercise-fitness/tricep-stretches

Cronkleton, E. (2019b, July 29). How and When to Include Static Stretching in Your Workout. Healthline; Healthline Media. https://www.healthline.com/health/exercise-fitness/static-stretching

Cronkleton, E. (2019c, September 9). What Is Neck Flexion? Plus Exercises for Improving Your Range of Motion. Healthline; Healthline Media. https://www.healthline.com/health/neck-flexion

Cummings Houdyshell, S. (2018). 10 Minute Full Body Resistance Band Stretch [YouTube Video]. In YouTube. https://www.youtube.com/watch?v=abqZwzk5LSw

CWT, D. R., MSPT, COMT, CFT. (2020, May 28). Best Yoga Poses for Sciatica Relief. Spine-Health. https://www.spine-health.com/blog/best-yoga-poses-sciatica-relief

Daisy. (2015a, March 11). Forward Leg Swings | Illustrated Exercise Guide. SPOTEBI. https://www.spotebi.com/exercise-guide/forward-leg-swings

Daisy. (2015b, March 12). Ankle Circles | Illustrated Exercise Guide. SPOTEBI. https://www.spotebi.com/exercise-guide/ankle-circles

Daisy. (2015c, March 12). Shoulder Rolls | Illustrated Exercise Guide. SPOTEBI. https://www.spotebi.com/exercise-guide/shoulder-rolls

Davis, K. (2020, April 9). 4 Types of Exercise Bands and How to Use Them. Health Perch. https://www.northwestpharmacy.com/healthperch/4-types-of-exercise-bands-and-how-to-use-them

Dynamic chest stretch | Exercise Videos & Guides. (n.d.). Bodybuilding.com. Retrieved September 3, 2022, from https://www.bodybuilding.com/exercises/dynamic-chest-stretch

Effects of Aging - OrthoInfo - AAOS. (2009). Aaos.org. https://orthoinfo.aaos.org/en/staying-healthy/effects-of-aging/

Evergreen, B. (2020, September 11). Why You Shouldn't Foam Roll Your IT Band? Evergreen Rehab and Wellness Coquitlam, Surrey and Langley. https://evergreenclinic.ca/why-you-shouldnt-foam-roll-your-it-band-what-to-do/

Exercise Right. (2016, October 18). What is resistance stretching and how do I do it? Exercise Right. https://exerciseright.com.au/what-is-resistance-stretching-and-how-do-i-do-it

Gaiam. (n.d.). 9 Foam Roller Dos and Don'ts. Gaiam. Retrieved September 5, 2022, from https://www.gaiam.com/blogs/discover/9-foam-roller-dos-and-don-ts

Getting specific: foam rolling and the foot. (n.d.). Human Kinetics Canada. Retrieved September 5, 2022, from https://canada.humankinetics.com/blogs/excerpt/getting-specific-foam-rolling-and-the-foot

Goldman, R. (2014, August 21). Ballistic Stretching: Is It Safe? Healthline. https://www.healthline.com/health/ballistic-stretching-it-safe

Harvard Health Publishing. (2019). Six tips for safe stretches - Harvard Health. Harvard Health; Harvard Health. https://www.health.harvard.edu/staying-healthy/six-tips-for-safe-stretches

Health Benefits of Stretching for Older Adults. (2019, June 29). LifeSpanFitness. https://canada.lifespanfitness.com/blogs/news/health-benefits-of-stretching-for-older-adults?shpxid=8ae7ff67-af87-47a7-ae1a-20cdb31cdcdc

Health Direct. (2018, October 18). Healthdirect Australia. Healthdirect.gov.au; Healthdirect Australia. https://www.healthdirect.gov.au/

Heitz, D., & Cirino, E. (2021, October 28). Sciatica Exercises: 6 Stretches for Pain Relief. Healthline. https://www.healthline.com/health/back-pain/sciatic-stretches

How Sitting All Day Affects Your Body -. (2020, September 22). The Vein Center of Florida & South Baldwin. https://veincenterofflorida.com/how-sitting-all-day-affects-your-body/

How To Do Back Extensions (Form & Benefits). (2022, January 13). Steel Supplements. https://steelsupplements.com/blogs/steel-blog/how-to-do-back-extensions-form-benefits

Jeffrey, P. (2015, February 9). Stretch Before Exercise? Not So Fast. | BU Today. Boston University. https://www.bu.edu/articles/2015/stretch-before-exercise-not-so-fast/

Kutcher, M. (2019, July 1). Regaining Flexibility After 60 | A Step by Step Guide. More Life Health - Seniors Health & Fitness. https://morelifehealth.com/articles/regaining-flexibility-guide

Lateral Flexion (Side Bend) Is The Best Lower Back Pain Treatment. (n.d.). Pilates Fitness. Retrieved August 30, 2022, from https://pilatesfitness.com.sg/lateral-flexion-side-bend-best-lower-back-pain-treatment/

Malacoff, J. (2018, May 24). 5 Signs You Need to Strengthen Your Upper Back | Fitness | MyFitnessPal. MyFitnessPal Blog. https://blog.myfitnesspal.com/5-signs-you-need-to-strengthen-your-upper-back/

Martins, N. (2019, November 12). Muscle Recovery: Essential to Your Next Workout. H.V.M.N. https://hvmn.com/blogs/blog/training-muscle-recovery-essential-to-your-next-workout

MasterClass. (2022, February 18). 8 Hip Flexor Stretches: How to Stretch Your Hip Flexors. MasterClass. https://www.masterclass.com/articles/hip-flexor-stretch

Mayo Clinic. (2018a). How do exercise and arthritis fit together? Mayo Clinic. https://www.mayoclinic.org/diseases-conditions/arthritis/in-depth/arthritis/art-20047971

Mayo Clinic. (2018b). Sciatica - symptoms and causes. Mayo Clinic. https://www.mayoclinic.org/diseases-conditions/sciatica/symptoms-causes/syc-20377435

Mayo Clinic. (2018c). What you need to know about exercise and chronic disease. Mayo Clinic. https://www.mayoclinic.org/healthy-lifestyle/fitness/in-depth/exercise-and-chronic-disease/art-20046049

Merriam-Webster. (2022). Merriam-Webster Dictionary. Merriam-Webster.com; Merriam-Webster. https://www.merriam-webster.com/

Mihailovich, K. (2021, March 2). 8 Easy Resistance Band Exercises for Seniors from an Occupational Therapist - Expert Fitness Supply. Expert Fitness Supply.

https://expertfitnesssupply.com/2021/03/02/8-easy-resistance-band-exercises-for-seniors-from-an-occupational-therapist/

Nast, C. (2017, December 20). 8 Foam Rolling Moves to Release Tight Spots From Head to Toe. SELF. https://www.self.com/story/foam-rolling-moves-release-tight-spots

Nast, C. (2020, August 4). 5 Post-Workout Stretches That Will Loosen Up Your Tight Muscles. SELF. https://www.self.com/gallery/post-workout-stretches

Padgett, A. (2019, November 11). How to Create the Ultimate Stretching Routine for Chronic Pain. Augusta Pain Center. https://augustapaincenter.com/create-ultimate-stretching-routine-chronic-pain/

Pedemonte, S. (n.d.). Upper Back Stretches. Your House Fitness. https://www.yourhousefitness.com/blog/upper-back-stretches

Pletcher, P. (2014, August 14). 5 Seated Back Pain Stretches for Seniors. Healthline. https://www.healthline.com/health/back-pain/stretches-for-seniors

Posture of the Month: Cat/Cow Pose. (2019, February 26). Your Pace Yoga. https://yourpaceyoga.com/blog/cat-cow/

Roberts, C. (2019, October 21). Stretching before or after a workout: Only one of them is right. CNET. https://www.cnet.com/health/fitness/stretch-before-or-after-a-work-which-is-best/

Rotman, C. (2021, September 7). 10 Best Stretches for Your Whole Body After a Workout - Circuit. Circuitliving.com. https://circuitliving.com/10-best-stretches-for-your-whole-body-after-a-workout/

Runyon, J. (2021, October 5). Leg swings (front to back) Movement Tutorial | MoveWellTM. Movewellapp.com. https://movewellapp.com/movements/leg-swings-front-to-back

Schirm, M. (2021, December 21). The 7 Best Dynamic Arm Stretches to Improve Your
Mobility and Warm Up for Exercise. LIVESTRONG.COM. https://www.livestrong.
com/article/354369-dynamic-arm-stretches/

Schrift, D. (n.d.). Ankle Stretching for Seniors and the Elderly – ELDERGYM®.
Eldergym.com. https://eldergym.com/ankle-stretching/

Schrift, D. (2019). Benefits of Stretching For Seniors And The Elderly – Eldergym®
Senior Fitness. Eldergym.com. https://eldergym.com/benefits-of-stretching/

Sears, B. (2022, February 22). The Easiest Exercise to Improve the Way Your Back
Bends Forward. Verywell Health. https://www.verywellhealth.com/low-back-
flexion-exercise-2696191

Seniorliving.org. (2022, May 24). Workouts & Exercises for Seniors | Senior Posture,
Flexibility, Strength & Diet. SeniorLiving.org. https://www.seniorliving.org/life/
active-senior/exercise/

Seniors and Pain Relief: Should I Be Foam Rolling? (2017, May 9). Life Enriching
Communities. https://lec.org/blog/seniors-and-pain-relief-should-i-be-foam-
rolling/

SET, S. F. (2022, March 28). 10 Best Chest Stretches for Before & After Workouts.
SET for SET. https://www.setforset.com/blogs/news/chest-stretches

Shoulder Blade Squeeze | Arthritis NSW. (2019, November 18). Www.arthritisnsw.org.
au. https://www.arthritisnsw.org.au/exercise-shoulder-blade-squeeze

SMR Pectorals Foam Roll. (2018, March 14). Adventure Performance Training. https://
adventureperformancetraining.com/smr-pectorals-foam-roll

Sullivan, C. (2021, July 21). 6 Benefits of Cobra Pose. Healthline. https://www.
healthline.com/health/fitness/benefits-of-cobra-pose

Toates, S. (2016, December 13). Cobra exercise for Sciatica | Chiropractor | Jersey | Dynamic Health. Dynamic Health, Jersey Chiropractor. https://dynamichealth. je/2016/12/13/cobra-exercise-for-sciatica

Umana, X. (2021, November 15). Senior Citizens and Stretching: What Are the Best Tips? Elite Care at Home Miami. https://www.miamielitecare.com/senior-citizens-and-stretching-what-are-the-best-tips/

Wade, P. (2021, March 22). Signs you're not stretching enough. The Independent. https://www.independent.co.uk/life-style/health-and-families/hiit-underbelly-b1820601.html

Walking Knee Hugs. (n.d.). Black Belt Wiki. Retrieved September 3, 2022, from https://blackbeltwiki.com/walking-knee-hugs

Warm Up Exercises for Seniors: Types + Why Seniors Should Do Them -. (2021, February 17). Seniors Mobility. https://seniorsmobility.org/exercises/warm-up-exercises-for-seniors/

Warm-up and cool-down. (2020, April 30). Www.nhsinform.scot. https://www. nhsinform.scot/healthy-living/keeping-active/before-and-after-exercise/warm-up-and-cool-down

Weatherspoon, D. (2020, February 24). Foam Roller for Back: 6 Exercises to Relieve Tightness and Pain. Healthline. https://www.healthline.com/health/roller-foam-for-back

What Are the Benefits of Torso Rotation Exercise? (n.d.). Fitness Together. Retrieved September 2, 2022, from https://fitnesstogether.com/weston-waltham/blog/what-are-the-benefits-of-torso-rotation-exercise-

Why Flexibility Is So Significant As We Age. (2019, April 27). Www. uniquehealthandfitness.com. https://www.uniquehealthandfitness.com/why-flexibility-is-so-significant-as-we-age

Why Stretch - 6 Short and Long Term Benefits to Make you Reach for your Stretch. (n.d.). RUHE. Retrieved August 31, 2022, from http://www.theruhe.com/blog/why-stretch-6-short-and-long-term-benefits-to-make-you-reach-for-your-stretch

Wrist flexor stretch. (2000, January 1). Best Health Magazine Canada. https://www.besthealthmag.ca/article/wrist-flexor-stretch/

Zaban, S. (n.d.). Exercise Tutorial: Lying Pec Stretch. Your House Fitness. Retrieved September 6, 2022, from https://www.yourhousefitness.com/blog/exercise-tutorial-lying-pec-stretch

Made in the USA
Las Vegas, NV
16 January 2024

84451493R00079